To 1
Ch

A beautiful person, both inside and out
who I was blessed to find
and
who has always loved me and believed in me,
even when I didn't.

"Accept what is,

Let go of what was,

and have faith in what will be."

Preface

In my back yard next to my deck is a small Laurel Oak tree that is overshadowed by a monstrous Live Oak tree. I first noticed this scrawny Laurel Oak when we visited the house while looking to move here over a decade ago. Since then, I have watched this Laurel Oak bravely and relentlessly scratch and claw it's way out from under the menacing Live Oak in an attempt to capture every slither of sunshine that it can possibly absorb in order to just stay alive. Because of its location, the small tree only has branches growing off of its left side, since the right side is butted up against its massive encroaching neighbor. The smaller tree can't exist as easily as other trees do because it always has something beyond its control trying to impede its very survival.

I tell you this because the small Laurel Oak reminds me of myself since I am someone with Parkinson's disease. Every day, the Laurel Oak has to fight for what it gets- just like us- and every day, it has opposition from something bigger than it is that is unrelenting, trying, just as hard, to take it out.

Unlike most people that you see walking about who don't have to worry about this horrible disease, Parkinson's patients have to endure a struggle every day, month-after-month, year-after-year. We go through each day doing everything we can to resist the effects of this disease as it tries its best to overpower us and rob us of our quality of life. We may not talk about it all the time, but that doesn't mean that it isn't always in the back of our minds, whether we want it to be there or not. We know it isn't hiding.

Every new day, we get up and we start this brave battle all over again. We know not to give in to it because it's always there. It's like Arnold Schwarzenegger in the movie The Terminator: "It can't be bargained with, it can't be reasoned with, it doesn't feel pity or remorse or fear, and it absolutely will not stop...EVER!"

Okay, so who am I and why do I feel as if I might be qualified to write a book about Parkinson's disease? Well, to start with, I need to tell you who I'm not. I want to make it known to everyone that I'm not a doctor. I'm also not a scientist actively looking for a cure (although I wish I could somehow contribute more to finding one). But I am a husband and a father who has a vested interest in learning as much about this disease as possible, which is exactly what I try to do.

Even though I'm not a doctor, I feel like I have a lot to bring to the table because unlike the doctors that I've seen who have only read about Parkinson's or seen it's effects in their patients, like you, I actually have first-hand knowledge about it because I live with it day-in-and-day-out. Unfortunately, we, as patients, don't have the luxury of being able to turn off thinking about it once we're off work. In the beginning, I fixated on my disease every waking moment, which was not a good idea. That's not to say that doctors are insensitive or don't care because that's certainly not the case at all. I'm extremely thankful for all the doctors I've ever been involved with. Where would we be without them?

I've been lucky enough in regards that I've never met a single doctor who wasn't completely focused on trying to help me any way they could that would improve my health as much as possible. I loved my previous doctor (kudos, Dr. Mayville!), but when she moved I had to find my current doctor who took over and has continued to do great things for me (kudos, Dr. Silver!). I'm saying that when it comes to Parkinson's, we, as patients, have a bit of an edge because we have personal experience with this disease and that gives us just a little more insight than our doctors have. Believe me, I would never bash doctors and all the good they do for us so please don't think that.

I should also say that this book is not a lone effort; it was written with the help of my wife and best friend, Charity. She's the reason I found my current doctor and the reason why my condition has improved so radically since being diagnosed. My wife is a truly amazing person. She's also one of the most intelligent people I know. I don't know how I was so lucky to find her, but I'm so thankful that I did because she has made my life so much happier and this challenging journey so much easier.

She was able to make such a large contribution to my health not only because of her compassion and natural caring attitude, but also because of her background. She has a degree in journalism, which she has effectively applied to helping me find the answers that I needed on a wide variety of topics. She's worked at CNN, had her own TV show on a local cable station where she did everything from editing, to producing and even anchored and worked on "Lawmakers", a show that featured state government. She's also written hundreds of articles for the local newspapers, had her work published in magazines, worked at the State Capitol and is now a published author and successful business owner, so she knows how to thoroughly investigate a subject to find the needed answers.

Since day one, my wife has immersed herself into learning as much as she can and has been relentless in her research so we can both learn everything we can get our hands on. Her instinct for digging up the facts has changed my life. I don't know what I would have done without her. I do know I wouldn't be nearly as far along with my treatment if it weren't for her.

But back to the book. I wrote the free guide "12 things you need to ask your doctor when you're diagnosed with Parkinson's" because I remember what it was like to hear the news that I had Parkinson's and not know the right questions to ask. Even though I had my wife by my side through all of this, I couldn't help but feel somewhat alone because it seemed as if this was *my* illness- not anyone else's. No matter how much support and love you're given, you still realize that, in the course of things, *you* are going to be the one to feel the symptoms; *you* are going to be the one to have to endure the medication and their side effects; *you* are going to have to be the one who has to alter their lifestyle. But while keeping it bottled up inside might be a noble thought, it isn't healthy, as I soon found out.

If you're like me, you also worried about how this disease was going to affect your family and the hardships and adjustments that they might have to make because of it. I didn't want to put them through all that, but when you're diagnosed, you don't have a choice so knowing that your family can be there and give you so much support is so reassuring. Even if you don't have family close by, you can still rely on your friends to help you through this.

I was fortunate enough to be surrounded by a loving spouse and family that cared, but I still couldn't help but to feel a little bit alone. That was my own fault. I was trying to retain ownership of my disease as much as possible so it didn't affect anyone else any more than was absolutely necessary. Looking back now, I see that this was a huge mistake because the one thing we all need during this time is support from others. I didn't want anyone else to have to feel that so I created a Facebook group to help others. The goal was to help them cope with what was happening to them like I was learning to cope with it.

There's a reason why I named my Facebook group **"Life With Parkinson's"** instead of "Existing With Parkinson's". Because it *is* all about living, and *not* just existing. Anyone can *exist* without even trying, but it takes something special in a person for them to actually *live,* especially when they have a debilitating condition constantly trying to knock them back down.

Oh, and one more thing - throughout this book, I'll periodically cover **"the 14 things (insights) I wish I had known when I was first diagnosed".** The purpose of this list is to prepare you ahead of time so you don't end up making the same mistakes that I did.

I don't claim to have all the answers (I wish I did and then this book would be much shorter) but I am learning more every day and I do have a lot to share with anyone who's willing to listen. If I can prevent others from repeating my mistakes and wasting unnecessary energy, time, effort and worry, then I've accomplished what I've set out to do.

Chapter 1

10.11.12

Right about now, you're probably wondering what the above numbers represent. Well, like every person living with Parkinson's, it represents a very important milestone in my life: it happens to be the day I was diagnosed. I didn't plan for my diagnosis date to be in-sync like that; it just so happened to turn out that way. It's actually pretty cool.

That Thursday in October was just supposed to be another regular day of me getting some answers to questions about what I was feeling. I didn't have any serious expectations and wasn't really overly-concerned about my doctor's appointment. In fact, in my mind, I had already expected to be told that it was just a part of growing older and that I needed to lose weight, clean up my eating and start taking better care of myself (blah, blah, blah). Y'know, the usual stuff a doctor tells you that you already know you should be doing, but that you never quite get around to actually doing until it's forced upon you. But never, in my wildest dreams, did I expect him to say what he said.

This doctor was the second neurologist that I had seen. Four months earlier, I had finally had enough and decided I needed to see a specialist because my symptoms weren't getting any better. Back then, I only had occasional tremors, they were only in my left hand, they were mild and they usually only happened when I wasn't exerting myself in some way. But even so, I still wasn't alarmed because I knew in my own mind that I had already figured it out; I just needed confirmation so I could move on.

That first doctor had examined me, had me do the typical slap-your-hands-on-your-legs and walk-up-and-down-the-hall evaluation and said I had the beginnings of essential tremors, which I didn't really believe. There was a parent of one of my son's friends who had essential tremors and I knew that mine were nothing like his so I blew off the diagnosis. I just thought he was guessing without taking all the facts into consideration because if he had seen the guy that I knew, he'd see that our symptoms were nothing alike.

At first, *I* thought my mild tremors were because of low blood sugar issues. To be honest, I was only going to a neurologist because my wife had made me. As far as I was concerned, it was a big waste of time because I already knew what was wrong. It was blood sugar- plain and simple. Anyone who saw what I ate on a daily basis would probably have been inclined to agree with me.

It made perfect sense to me because the shaking didn't happen all the time and I'll have to admit, I wasn't exactly the picture of health. In fact, I was really abusing sugar in so many ways. I ate pretty much everything but the furniture, specializing in a lot of fast food and as much chocolate as I could possibly get my hands on. But the most abusive way I was hurting myself was from drinking sweet tea.

Being raised in the South, I grew up loving sweet tea. I had consistently drunk sweet tea since I was a kid. And it didn't qualify as sweet tea unless you could almost stand a spoon upright in the glass because of the high sugar content. But although I had been hooked on it all of my life, I was now drinking more of it than ever. In fact, I was routinely going through about a gallon of it every day. You read that right: *a gallon.* Since I was using about two cups of sugar per gallon, I was getting way too much sugar on a daily basis. So I planted the blood sugar idea in my head because I knew I had it coming after abusing sugar for so many years.

My sugar theory also made sense because both of my parents had been type 2 diabetics with my mom having been on insulin. Statistics show that if both parents are diabetic, their child's risk of also being diabetic are 1 in 2, so the odds were already stacked against me. Add that to the fact that I was middle-aged, considered obese and had a sedentary lifestyle and red flags were being thrown up all over the place. I could have easily been the poster child for pre-diabetes. Besides, everyone knows that mild tremors are a classic sign of low blood sugar- especially for someone who was pre-diabetic, which I had also been diagnosed as being not long before. Anyway, that was what I was expecting to hear.

Boy, was I wrong.

The doctor didn't even ask me about sugar. In fact, he never even brought up the subject of diabetes, at all. I kept thinking "this guy doesn't know what he's doing". *Hello? I'm overweight! I eat sugar by the buckets! What is it with everyone asking me to alternate slapping my hands back and forth against my leg? Why are you watching me walk up and down the hall? Where exactly did you go to medical school?*

I had already told him that I had seen another neurologist (also at the request of my wife). He asked me what the first doctor had told me and I said I would tell him after he examined me. So he had me do all of the usual movements and made all his little notes. Finally, when the appointment was over, he looked at me and said: "So the other doctor told you it was Parkinson's, right?"

What?!

I just sat there. I know I must have had a stunned look on my face. It was like time froze all of a sudden. I remember sitting there thinking *you're wrong! I have diabetes! Diabetes!! Where did you get Parkinson's? I'm too young to have that!* The concept of Parkinson's had never, ever even crossed my mind. Surely, this guy must be wrong. I didn't know any better so I was secretly hoping that Parkinson's was just another fancy name for essential tremors (I didn't know anything about Parkinson's, but at this point, I was still holding out hope that the two were one and the same). Here's how the conversation went:

"*Parkinson's?*"

"Parkinson's."

"Are you sure?"

"I'm ninety-nine percent sure."

"Are you sure it isn't the beginnings of essential tremors?"

"No. It's Parkinson's. Is that what the other doctor told you?"

"Yeah. He said it looked like essential tremors."

"Well, maybe back then it looked like essential tremors, but now, it looks like Parkinson's."

And that was how I learned I had Parkinson's.

I hadn't brought my wife with me to the appointment because I didn't think I needed to. After all, it wasn't anything to worry about. It was going to be another routine appointment where the doctor was going to chew me out for not taking better care of myself. I had heard the same rhetoric for years from other doctors. I had no reason to believe that this one was going to be any different.

Before I could get out to my car in the parking lot and call my wife, my hands were shaking (and not from the Parkinson's, either). When I finally managed to force out the words, needless to say she was as shocked as I was. It was less than six miles to my house, but it still felt like it took forever to drive it. I walked in the door, walked over to my wife, we hugged and we both started crying.

It was then that I realized I had only seen what I wanted to see. We sat down and immediately started searching online for "Parkinson's disease" so we would know what we were up against. After reading up on it and looking back, we both realized that I had been experiencing symptoms for years that we hadn't associated with the disease. We never made the connection to Parkinson's because we didn't know how to do that or what to look for.

I'll be the first to admit that before I was diagnosed, I didn't really know anything about Parkinson's, either. But as determined as I was on October 11, 2012 to prove that I didn't have essential tremors, I still would have gladly taken that over Parkinson's. Unfortunately, it wasn't up to me.

Once I calmed down, I was confused and I had so many questions. So I spent the next few weeks doing what any hard-headed person in my position who didn't want to hear the truth would do: I got a second opinion.

And then a third.

And then a fourth.

And then a fifth.

And then a sixth.

My logic was simple: I figured if I went to enough doctors, eventually I was bound to find someone who would tell me something different, or, in other words, tell me what I *wanted* to hear instead of the truth. That was my way of dealing with denial. As far as I was concerned, it was a foolproof plan. But guess what? It didn't happen the way I wanted because I actually *did* have Parkinson's.

Every Parkinson's patient remembers the day they were first diagnosed because that was the day their life changed forever. It's like you're traveling along in a normal lifeline and suddenly you have to veer off and go in a different direction because you now have something new that you're being forced to take into consideration, whether you like it or not. Something very scary.

Anyone who has ever been diagnosed with Parkinson's will tell you that you can't help but be flooded with so many emotions all at once: fear, curiosity, sadness and maybe even resentment and anger. It's completely natural to go through this phase because you have so many questions and you don't know what to expect, what to ask and who to ask. But the thing is you can't allow those emotions to control your life and they will- if you give them the chance.

Just because you have Parkinson's doesn't mean that your life has to be based off of the fear that it generates. Fear isn't going to make it go away. It isn't going to help you improve your health or your quality of life. It isn't going to have any positive contribution whatsoever. What it will do is consume you and bring you down much faster by leading to more stress and more worry than you deserve to go through. And as we'll discuss later, stress doesn't go well with Parkinson's.

I'll be the first to admit that finding out you have Parkinson's is a shock. Actually, that's being simplistic. To say that it's a shock is a massive understatement. The truth is it's downright frightening because you don't know what to think. Your first reaction is to be scared of the unknown. You automatically think about our own mortality and you can't help but worry about what will happen to you and how quickly it will happen. That might not be a healthy way of thinking, but it's what you're left with.

I'm one of those people who believe that everything happens for a reason. Developing Parkinson's is no exception. Is this what I would have wanted for myself? Absolutely not. But it's here and I know I have to deal with it or it will take me over.

I wouldn't wish Parkinson's on anyone. But I have to accept it for what it is and move on. In the beginning I wanted to be angry. I wanted to feel hurt. I wanted to feel sorry for myself. I wanted to lash out at destiny and scream "WHY ME?!" But honestly, as much as I would have loved to do just that none of it would have made me feel any better. And it certainly wasn't going to help my situation. It was nothing more than a waste of my time and energy- neither of which I could spare for such nonsense.

As much as I would rather not have Parkinson's, I accept the fact that I do and I move on. I have to believe that there's a reason behind it. For almost three years, I didn't know what that reason was.

Now, I do.

I believe that I developed this horrible disease so I could use my experience to help others who have also been diagnosed. That's why

I started my Facebook group. That's why I chose to write this book. And that's why I'll continue to do whatever I can to talk to as many people and offer as much assistance as I can. I didn't know what to do when I was diagnosed and I spent a lot of time and effort doing the wrong things. I spent a lot of time being frustrated and anxious to learn the truth. I worried and fixated on all of the negative and let that control my thinking. I don't want anyone else to go through that unnecessarily.

I'll admit, there are days when it hits me more than others and when it's one of those days, I have a hard time with it. But when I experience one of those times, I think back to a saying I read a long time ago. For many years, it never really resonated with me because, let's face it, we often ignore how good we have things until they aren't so good anymore. Forgive me for not remembering who said it and I may not be quoting the exact original phrase, but it goes something like this:

> *"I complained because I had no shoes, until I met a man who had no feet."*

What a powerful statement! It reminds us that as bad as things are and as hopeless as we think they might look, we still need to be thankful for what we have. We might have it bad (or, at least *our* perception of bad), but in the long run there are always others who would gladly trade their situation for ours in a heartbeat.

Being diagnosed might have changed the direction I was taking in my life, but it didn't mean that I had stop moving forward altogether. I knew my life wasn't over just because of a stupid disease. I wasn't going to let that happen. That isn't fair to me, my wife or my kids. It's important for every Parkinson's patient to know that, which brings us to the first thing I wish I had known when I was first diagnosed:

Insight #1: Your life isn't over.

If you get nothing else from this book, at least remember that. You can't start out your treatment worried about things that haven't even happened. Sure, you're going to be scared. It's something new to you. It's the unknown. You won't understand it. And as humans, we always fear what we don't understand. That's to be expected. But you can't let it run your life, which it will if you let it. You can't let it dictate what you do and you certainly can't let it determine how you live.

Your life *isn't* over- not by a long shot. In fact, you need to know that you can live a full life as long as you're willing to make the necessary changes to help make that happen. Your life doesn't have to be cut short just because you have Parkinson's. You have a huge impact on how well the rest of your life plays out. Will you have to experience certain things that other people without Parkinson's don't ever have to experience? Of course you will. It goes with the territory. But just because you have this disease doesn't mean you should give up, crawl in the corner and let life pass you by. There's absolutely no reason why you shouldn't plan on living just the same as you would if you didn't have Parkinson's.

I know there'll be challenges, there'll be setbacks and there'll be obstacles. I get that. But instead of automatically giving in to defeat I choose to look at it this way: life is full of challenges. This just happens to be one that I have to focus a little more attention on than most others.

Now you know the significance of 10.11.12 in my life and how things were never the same from that day forward. That set of numbers is forever stuck in my mind. Do you remember *your* diagnosis date?

Symptoms I Missed (and you might, too!)

As my wife and I began to immerse ourselves in learning as much as we could about Parkinson's, we both realized that we had missed key symptoms that pointed directly to Parkinson's disease that had been happening to me for the past few years and we didn't even know it. That's the crazy thing about Parkinson's: you could be experiencing telltale signs for quite some time and never put two-and-two together.

As near as I could tell, my first symptoms had started between 4 and 5 years earlier. The first symptom I could pinpoint as being Parkinson's-related was insomnia. Out of the blue, and for no apparent reason that I could ever put a cause to, I started having trouble sleeping. I'm talking about a person that had slept like a baby for 45 years and now, all of a sudden, I was waking up 6 to 8 times a night, every night- sometimes more than that. I could lie in bed for 8 or 9 hours and still wake up exhausted the next morning because I was never getting restful sleep.

I would visit doctor after doctor, some that my wife and I researched on our own and others that were recommended to me. Each one seemed to want to help, but the appointment always ended in the same manner: take a pill. But I had a couple of real problems with this suggestion. For one thing, I had gone my entire life without having to take medication so it was a little overwhelming for me to suddenly be told that I needed medicine just to help hold myself together. My second problem with this logic was that I knew I wasn't suffering from a medication deficiency, so why did I need it now? This is the one time when I get aggravated at the medical community for treating the symptom and *not* the cause.

Despite my hesitation, I was so desperate to get good, quality sleep that I succumbed and took the medication that they gave me. Some made me feel like a zombie (even the following day) while others did nothing. Besides, I knew I didn't want to have to rely on a pill to get some sleep (correction: I *wasn't* going to rely on a pill to get some sleep). Long story short, I continued to have sleeping issues.

Another symptom that I never made the connection to Parkinson's was depression. Now, I'll admit, I have always been laid-back and easy-going, but when the depression started setting in I couldn't have cared less about what was going on around me. I wanted to, but I could barely force myself to care about much of anything. I began to abandon regular bathing; I wore old, worn clothing all the time and never cared to leave the house. I never cared to put the effort into it. Emotionally, I was a wreck.

In January of 2011, I started noticing that my left hand would shake slightly when I picked up a drink. But since my right hand (my dominant hand) was as steady as a rock, I didn't think much of it. Why should I? I blamed it on my frozen shoulder acting up (I'll talk more about that later). The tremors stayed at that level until summer came when and they started getting a little worse, but still not what you would consider to be bad. That finally prompted me to go see the first neurologist. And the rest, as they say, was history.

Back To My Time-table...

After receiving my official diagnosis, and since I had a score of Parkinson's:1, Essential Tremors: 1, I needed a tie-breaker so I went to the third neurologist who examined me and confirmed that it was, in fact, Parkinson's. The fourth neurologist also agreed with that diagnosis. I would have been happy to stop at that point and utilize one of those doctors, but my wife, always looking for the best treatment options for me, found a movement disorder specialist down at Emory University in Atlanta, one of the most prestigious medical facilities anywhere around. Since Emory is a teaching hospital, I knew that the neurologists there would be cutting-edge, something I desperately wanted to take advantage of.

By this time, it was almost the end of 2011. So far, my tally was three doctors who agreed that it was Parkinson's. I wanted so much to be vindicated and prove them wrong, but by now I knew that that ship had sailed. All I was looking for now was answers- a lot of them.

As expected, the Emory doctor was young and well-versed on the latest treatments. But there was one problem that I really needed help with. I had noticed that my trunk would shake- especially when I was out in public. The more people that were around, the worse my stomach would vibrate. It got so noticeable and I became so self-conscious of it that I resorted to folding my arms across my chest in a feeble attempt to hide it from onlookers, but even that wasn't sufficient. I was so embarrassed that I finally curtailed my exposure to other people as much as possible. And it wasn't just reserved for acquaintances: it also happened around my extended family and even those in my own household.

When I asked my Emory doctor about it, his response was "I've never seen anything like that in a Parkinson's patient. I have no idea what that is." I decided to just ignore it, as if it were going to go away on it's own (which, of course, it didn't). What did it end up being caused by? Believe it or not, it was from nerves.

I had grown so accustomed to hiding my disease from everyone else that I unknowingly became super-protective of my secret. At this point, I had been officially diagnosed almost three months; yet, the only ones who knew were my immediate family. I didn't even bother to share it with my friends. I knew that it was only a matter of time before someone would pick up on the symptoms and figure it out for themselves, but I certainly wasn't in any kind of a hurry to help them. In the process of hiding from everyone, I was creating a huge amount of anxiety for myself. As if that wasn't bad enough, I was internalizing all of that anxiety, which manifested into the trembling in my trunk that the doctor was seeing.

My wife kept assuring me that it was okay to tell others that I had Parkinson's, but for some reason, I was ashamed to say anything. I felt as if someone would judge me for being less of a man so I continued to hide it. I just knew that others would think differently of me and would treat me differently because of the disease. But, the truth was, it was eating me up inside and causing me even worse symptoms. Finally, after much pleading from my wife for almost an entire year, I agreed that she could begin telling people, but only a select few of our closest friends to start with (I know it probably sounds ridiculous that I was so protective of my condition, but, believe me, it was a HUGE step for me just to do that).

After a few more months, and even more reassurance from my wife, I conceded and began to tell people of my disease. Then, a funny thing happened. The more people I told, the easier it became to talk about it. Not only that, but the severity of the trunk shaking started to diminish. Within the next few months, I was totally at ease with opening up about the subject and my trunk shaking was completely gone, which brings me to the second thing I wish I had known when I was first diagnosed:

Insight #2: It's important that you not be embarrassed to share your diagnosis with others.

The more people you open up to, the better you'll be able to handle it yourself. Not following that advice was the mistake I made. I shied away from opening up and speaking about it to anyone because I was afraid of so many things:

afraid others would look at me differently
afraid they would start to treat me differently
afraid they would smother me with sympathy
afraid that they would suddenly feel awkward being around me because they wouldn't know what to say and what not to say
afraid others would be afraid to bring up the subject because they wouldn't know how sensitive I was talking about it
afraid others (especially my friends) would avoid me, altogether.

I hoped that, somehow, if I didn't bring it up, those around me would never know, as if I could hide it for the rest of my life. But I was already sabotaging my efforts more by holding it in and trying to deal with it all by myself instead of accepting it for what it was and moving on. All the while I thought I was doing myself a favor, I was actually causing myself even more grief and making matters worse.

I spent my time believing that others wouldn't accept me for who I was. I convinced myself that I was damaged goods, that I could no longer contribute as much as I could have before. It was as if my value had suddenly plummeted the day I was diagnosed. In my heart, I knew that I would be looked upon as someone needy or handicapped.

But as soon as I began to open up, I found myself shocked. I learned that others didn't react that way to me- not one single time. My friends were still my friends and they supported me and treated me the same as they had always treated me. In fact, things were just the opposite of what I feared. They made it known that they were there for me even more than ever before. I realized that I didn't have anything to be afraid of. In fact, I wish I hadn't wasted so much time being stupid in my assumptions, none of which ever came true. It reminded me of the saying "most of the things you worry about never happen." How true that is.

The bad news is that since Parkinson's disease is progressive, our symptoms are guaranteed to get worse over time. Unfortunately, there's nothing you can do to change the direction of that course. The good news is that there's plenty you can do to *prolong* that journey as much as possible.

The rate at which your disease worsens depends largely on *you*. If you choose to ignore your symptoms, to do nothing and rely on your medication to do all the work, to sit back and anxiously hope and pray that someone comes up with a cure or, worse, to not accept the truth for what it is, like I tried to do in the beginning, you can be guaranteed that your symptoms will get worse much quicker than is necessary. But if you decide to take a stand and fight back with everything you can do to slow its progression, then you'll live a longer, happier and more productive life.

Like it or not, Parkinson's disease is here to stay. But it only has as much hold over our lives as we give it. You can either sit back, do nothing and let Parkinson's run your life into the ground right before your very eyes sooner than you could possibly imagine. Or, you can do something about it. If you fight back, kicking and screaming, you have the ability to make a huge difference.

It's all up to you.

Chapter 2

Some Basic (and Important) Things You Should Know About Parkinson's Disease

If you think about Parkinson's, you can't help but think about the two most famous people in our lifetime that have the disease: Michael J. Fox and Muhammad Ali. If there were a bright side to their diagnosis it would be that their celebrity status has brought a much greater awareness to the disease, of which we can all be thankful for. It also encouraged Fox to start the Michael J. Fox Foundation, which has been instrumental in bringing global awareness to the disease and has diligently sought to find a cure.

Through the years, we've all watched Fox and Ali battle this disease and the toll that it's taken on their lives. Ali might not have developed symptoms until later on in years (to this day, I still believe that his disease was brought on due to the physical abuse his head suffered as a result of his profession, since concussions are a risk factor), but Michael J. Fox didn't fit that mold.

In 1991, a then 29 year-old Fox was filming "Doc Hollywood" right outside of Gainesville, Florida (my hometown), when he noticed his first symptom: his pinkie finger began to tremble. Nowadays, when you see Fox, he's in a continuous fight just trying to keep his body still. Most people believe that they're witnessing the effects of the disease, when, in reality, what they're actually seeing more of is the effects of his medication as it tries to hold back his true Parkinson's symptoms.

Fox suffers from tremors due to a condition known as dyskinesia. It's actually ironic. The very medicine that he takes to control his disease causes dyskinesia, which causes tremors. He can't stop taking the medication because it is helping him in other ways so he has no choice but to live with the dyskinesia as the price he pays for not having tremors.

The general public also probably isn't aware that there are other famous people who share, or shared, our condition:

- Reverend Billy Graham
- Pope John Paul II
- "Peanuts" creator Charles Schultz
- Former Alabama Governor George Wallace
- Former U.S. Attorney General Janet Reno
- Maurice White (founder and lead singer of the musical group Earth, Wind and Fire)
- Singer Linda Ronstadt
- Singer Johnny Cash
- Roger Bannister (first person to run a four-minute mile and, coincidentally, a neurologist)
- Actress Estelle Getty (Golden Girls)
- Actress Deborah Kerr
- Actor Robin Williams
- Actor Bob Hoskins
- Comic/actor Billy Connolly
- Actor Vincent Price
- Radio personality Casey Kasem
- Adolf Hitler

If you randomly asked the general public what they knew about Parkinson's disease it's likely that almost everyone you encountered would have at least heard about it, if nothing else. If you went one step further and asked them to tell you what it was, you probably wouldn't find many who could tell you in-depth details about it, but chances are they could at least say it was a medical condition that caused a person to shake. They would probably also tell you that it was something that old people got. That's pretty much the extent of what they'd know. I'm ashamed to admit it, but to be honest, before I was diagnosed, I was part of this group. Like others, I knew nothing about Parkinson's because I didn't have a reason to know.

Then there would be a group of individuals who had heard of the disease, but really had no idea what it was or anything about it. These people usually remain in the dark about it unless it happens to hit them or someone who is close to them, forcing them to learn more about it strictly because of circumstances.

But those with Parkinson's know just how erroneous this portrayal of the disease is. We know that it has to do with a lot more than just shaking and we also know that it isn't only confined to older people. In fact, it's important to realize that there are a lot of things newly-diagnosed people probably don't know about Parkinson's, but, for their own sake, need to know.

How Parkinson's Disease Occurs In The First Place

It sounds a little bit simplistic to just say that Parkinson's is due to dopamine-producing neurons in the brain dying off. That sums up the end result, but it doesn't say anything about what precedes that action. A better question would be: "*how* and *why* do these neurons die off in the first place?

We all walk around not ever thinking about the number of neurons we have in our brains, seemingly unaware and completely uninterested. It isn't a concern for us because there's no reason for it to be. That is, until we realize that we have a degenerative disease that's directly affecting our brain. It's something that we take for granted until we're given a reason to no longer ignore its importance. Now, all of a sudden, the preservation of neurons has catapulted itself into being the single most important thing in our lives and we realize that it not only drives the very direction of our lives, but the quality of it, too.

When a patient is diagnosed with Parkinson's disease, they believe that they still have the "normal" amount of neurons in their brain. And why wouldn't they? They have no reason to believe that they shouldn't. But then, your Parkinson's diagnosis surfaces and now you're told that that underlying issue that has never been a problem before is suddenly not only an issue, but a really big deal that is going to impact and change your life forever.

Unfortunately, we have no idea how big of a deal it really is until we've been explained the "big picture". The fact of the matter is that by the time a patient is diagnosed with Parkinson's disease, they've already lost roughly a minimum of 50 to as much as 80 percent of their neurons- neurons that we'll never get back. So holding on to those precious few remaining ones quickly becomes priority number one. The fact that brain cells have been quietly dying off for quite some time- even years and possibly even for a decade or more before your disease is given an identity, is known as a "pre-symptomatic disease" because it has been occurring long before you began to notice symptoms. It's scary to think that you went years not realizing that something wasn't right.

If you could somehow keep the remaining neurons that you have then this would be the end of the story and it could all be chalked up to a simple maintenance routine. But it's not that simple. You see, your neurons continue to die off, regardless of what we do and there's nothing we can do to stop that from happening. If there were treatments available that could accomplish that, every Parkinson patient would gladly take advantage of them. But what we *can* do is incorporate certain "disease-modifying treatments" that *slows down* that loss as much as possible.

But Parkinson's disease doesn't just randomly occur. It can also occur because of the influence of other factors outside of our brain. One that is drawing considerable criticism from, believe it or not, chemical manufacturers, is the notion that pesticides can cause Parkinson's. At the time of this writing, chemical-making giant Monsanto has begun being slapped with lawsuits from workers who claim their cancer was caused from handling Monsanto's signature product, the weed killer Roundup. It should come as no surprise since scientists have been linking Parkinson's disease to pesticide exposure for years.

The sources of Parkinson's don't stop there. Researchers have found that taking certain types of psychiatric medications for extended periods of time have been shown to produce Parkinson's. The list of medications center around those prescribed to children who have been diagnosed with ADD or ADHD.

Then, there are some experts who believe that Parkinson's disease starts in the gut and spreads to the brain by way of an unlikely ally: the vagus nerve. The longest of the 12 cranial nerves, the vagus nerve extends from your brainstem all the way down to your abdomen, connecting with vital organs along the way- mainly your lungs and heart. It is the control center for the parasympathetic nervous system. Its duties involve communicating with every organ in the body and being involved with all of your unconscious bodily functions like the beating of your heart and the inhalation and expulsion of air from your lungs.

But sometimes, good things take a wrong turn. A recent study conducted by researchers from Aarhus University and Aarhus University Hospital in Denmark and published in the journal "Annals of Neurology", studied how the body could be using the vagus nerve as the premium highway to spread the damaging effects of Parkinson's from the gut up into the brain, where it can really do significant damage.

The connection dates back some 45 years when medical practitioners routinely performed a procedure known as a vagotomy, or the severance of the vagus nerve in the stomach, as a way to treat ulcers. The Aarhus team of researchers checked the registry of over 15,000 patients who had undergone the operation and what they found was interesting. It seems that after a 20-year period following the surgery, their risk of developing Parkinson's was half that of individuals who had not had the surgery. Coincidence?

Seeming to further substantiate this theory is the fact that so many newly-diagnosed Parkinson patients experienced digestive issues prior to their diagnosis. They believe that the connection between gastroenterologic pathology and neurologic pathology can be directly linked via the vagus nerve. Although more studies will have to be conducted, and if this is true, it does shed light on the possibility that an individual could substantially lower their risk of developing Parkinson's disease simply by taking better care of their digestive system and eating a clean, healthy diet.

What exactly is Parkinson's disease?

It's unfair to simply categorize Parkinson's as a disease where you shake. It's also unfair to downplay it as just another thing that you risk getting as you get older. It's called a progressive neurodegenerative disorder because it does progress in severity and the number of neurons does decline. There's nothing that you can do about either one occurring, but there is *a lot* that you can do about how *quickly* each one occurs. *That* is the part that you need to dwell on. Not the disease, itself, because there's nothing you can do to change that, but focusing, instead, on what you can do to fight back.

The neurons we're talking about produce the very important signaling chemical called dopamine. It's called a "signaling chemical" because that's exactly what it does: it signals the muscles to move. Those individuals without Parkinson's unknowingly take this action for granted because it's an involuntary action, meaning they don't have to give it any thought (just like all of us did before we were diagnosed). If they want to pick up a fork and feed themselves, they do it. If they want to tap a pencil in rhythm with a song on the radio, they're able to do it without wondering if they can. Parkinson patients can't.

The part of your brain that houses these vital dopamine neurons is called the substantia nigra, which is located just above the spinal cord. No one really understands why Parkinson's attacks and destroys these neurons, but it does and it does it very efficiently.

In order to dispel some of the rumors and falsehoods surrounding Parkinson's disease, I decided to answer the three most common questions that I've had people ask me. Chances are, you've heard them, too.

Fact #1: Parkinson's disease doesn't just affect older people.

It wasn't very long ago that a vast majority of people diagnosed with

Parkinson's were over the age of 60. Then, more and more people began being diagnosed at a younger age, say in their 50s and even their 40s, which spurred the need for the term "young onset Parkinson's". But even those guidelines have now changed.

There are currently about 1.5 million Americans who have been diagnosed with Parkinson's disease with between 7 and 10 million worldwide and another 60,00 Americans being added to the tally each year with that number expected to continue climbing. But even with that level of newly-diagnosed patients, only about 4 percent are under the age of 50. Still, the fact remains that Parkinson's is finding younger and younger victims.

There are even cases of teenagers getting Parkinson's disease. That's right: *teenagers.* I think the youngest I've read about was a 16-year old girl. As bad as it was for me to be diagnosed at 49, I couldn't imagine being told that at her age. Can you imagine being in the prime of your high school years looking at your life ahead of you and all of the possibilities and dreams that you're looking forward to and suddenly finding out that you have an "old person's disease" like Parkinson's?

It might be hard to comprehend, but whereas, in the past, it seemed that Parkinson's disease predominantly attacked older individuals, there are now an increasing number of cases of teenagers being diagnosed with it. This is no longer about an isolated case here and there. How is that possible? It's because of some of the things that we're exposed to from the world around us.

Scientists now understand just how many different factors there are that come into play to increase the likelihood that a person will develop Parkinson's disease (aside from the ones that I've already mentioned). They refer to these factors as "nature and nurture". "Nature" refers to our genes while "nurture" refers to the world around us.

When you talk about the nurture set of risk factors, you see that our lifestyle has a lot to do with the increased chances of contracting Parkinson's. One factor has to do with the toxic environment that we live in. When you refer to the environment, we're talking about everything that can contribute to the increased risk that isn't associated with genetics (nature). When you think about it, that's actually a very broad field of factors.

The Risk of Toxins

Our bodies are exposed to an extremely high level of toxins every single day that our grandparents, and even our parents, were never subjected to (or, at least if they were exposed to some of these toxins, it was in considerably smaller amounts). If you take into account all of the perfumes, chemicals, additives, preservatives, artificial this-and-that, dyes and plastics that we eat, groom with, bathe with, wear, eat our food from, cook our food in, store our food in or live in, it turns out to be a staggering number of ways we expose ourselves to these toxins that are anything but natural.

But it isn't just the things that we use that increase our risk. Research has also proven that people can develop Parkinson's just because of where they live. Rural farming areas that are sprayed with pesticides and herbicides are at an increased risk. Also at risk are the people who live near industrial areas that emit certain compounds into the atmosphere and into the surrounding soil and water supplies. The most common of these culprits are iron deposits, petroleum products, copper and manganese.

It used to be that seafood was touted as being one of the most healthy food sources you could incorporate into your diet, particularly because of the heart-healthy omega-3 fatty acids and other vital nutrients that it provided. Not anymore. Today, those individuals whose diet contains a larger percentage of seafood, predominantly shellfish, will also see a much higher risk of developing Parkinson's. This is due to the high levels of heavy metals, predominantly mercury, that are making their way into our rivers, streams and oceans, eventually ending up in the seafood that we eat.

Another problem is organic pollutants such as polychlorinated biphenyls, or PCBs. PCBs were first used in manufacturing back in

1929 when they were widely used for electrical insulation, as well as in lubricants, adhesives, inks, paints, flame-retardant products and even carbon-less copy paper. But it was soon realized that PCBs were detrimental to the health of those exposed to it, as well as being harmful to the environment. Even though their use was eventually banned, there are still traces of it to be found. Approximately ten percent of PCBs are still around today.

But just because you aren't exposed to these types of older products doesn't mean you're out of the woods. You can become exposed to PCBs from the incineration of municipal waste, which also releases other harmful compounds, including dangerous hydrogen chloride. PCBs can also make their way into your life by leaking out of old equipment into landfills and, eventually, out into the air. And PCBs can even be released into the atmosphere from contaminated bodies of water through natural evaporation.

Some studies have shown a connection between your occupation and the increased likelihood of developing Parkinson's. One of the most common of these professions is welders, because of the fact that metals are melted in order to be bonded together, which releases poisonous vapors. Those at risk also include individuals who handle or work with petroleum products or metals, such as industrial workers. It has also been shown that an increased number of farmers, and even recreational gardeners and nursery workers, are contracting Parkinson's. This is due to the vast array of pesticides, herbicides and insecticides that they are exposed to on a continuous basis.

I know about this last one first-hand because I grew up on a farm where we routinely used pesticides. Back then (we're talking some 35 years ago) no one knew anything about the long-term effects that handling these poisons could create. We never considered that there would be repercussions to our health because of the exposure. I spent years touching these products day-in-and-day-out without ever having access to fresh water to wash my hands. No one raised awareness about it and we certainly didn't know any better.

That was strike one against me.

Certain types of clothing can also up your chances of having Parkinson's, specifically those made from petroleum products to produce a water-tight seal, such as waders, gloves and raincoats, just to name a few. There has also been links between Parkinson's and clothing produced using chemicals that are designed to repel insects, such as mosquitoes. Lastly, people who experience some type of traumatic brain injury where the individual experiences a loss of consciousness or even amnesia which leads to inflammation within the brain see an increased risk, as well. Concussions top that list.

Fact #2: Genetics can play a huge part in whether or not you end up with Parkinson's.

As I mentioned before, when you talk about the "nature" side of risk factors, you're speaking of genetics. Research shows that men are more susceptible to contracting Parkinson's than are women, primarily because men are more likely to be found in occupations that expose them to contaminants, than are women.

Although the connection between genetics and Parkinson's is only around 10 percent, that still translates into 1 in every 10 patients. That might not sound like a high number until you consider the point that someone has to be that one person. In my case, that one person just happened to be me.

Here's a little background on genetic testing for Parkinson's without getting too technical. Back in 1997, researchers at the National Institutes of Health (NIH) discovered that when there were mutations in the SCNA gene, it coincided with an increased prevalence of Parkinson's. Seven years later, scientists discovered that the presence of mutation in yet another gene, LRRK2, also led to an increased risk of developing Parkinson's. Don't worry because this will all make sense in a minute.

All of us gather genes from both our father and our mother. When these genes are "normal", we can go through life without fear of Parkinson's through genetics. At that point, the only ways we will acquire the disease is if we fall into one of the categories that increase our chances of developing it, which are the environmental influences (nurture) or chance. The truth is, no one really knows why some people even get Parkinson's.

But let's say that we inherit a "bad" gene from our father. Now, our genetic risk of Parkinson's goes up slightly, but not too terribly much. Now, let's make matters even worse and become one of those people who are unfortunate enough to inherit a "bad" gene from both their father *and* their mother. Now, the odds are suddenly really stacked against you.

Still, even though you might have an increased risk on one or even both sides of you family, it doesn't *guarantee* that you're going to develop Parkinson's: it only means that your *risk* is increased.

I never thought about the connection genetics had with Parkinson's until some time after I found out about my situation. When I was a kid, I remember my maternal grandfather's left arm would shake constantly. We don't know whether or not his right arm was affected because he had only had his right arm from the elbow up. Believe it or not, he had lost the rest of it while dynamite fishing back around the turn of the twentieth century when it was still legal to do so where we lived. Back then, everyone called his condition "palsy". When I was diagnosed and began doing research, I discovered that palsy was what they used to call Parkinson's disease back in his day. Despite never being on any medication and never exercising, he lived to the ripe old age of 92 and ended up dying of pneumonia. That meant one genetic bad marker from my mother's side of the family.

My father died at age 81 from pulmonary fibrosis (PF). But, to our surprise, when we received the death certificate, the autopsy listed Parkinson's as the secondary diagnosis. We were so fixated on his treatment for PF that I never knew he had Parkinson's. That meant one genetic marker from my father's side of the family. So, now I had a close relative on my mother's side of the family *and* one on my father's side who had it. This was just one of the reasons why my risk of getting it went up even more, in addition to the pesticide exposure.

Strike two...

But just because you have a family history of Parkinson's doesn't mean that you're destined to get it, too. There are so many factors that come into play here. Even so, if you know of someone related to you that has it, it's better to get checked out sooner rather than later. If I had known at the time how much of a risk I was in, I would have looked into it more.

Initially, it might be discouraging for a young person to acquire an "old person's disease", but there is some good news for young-onset patients: they actually have their age working to their benefit. It seems that younger people don't develop the same type of Parkinson's as older people. Usually, the younger the patient is when diagnosed, the smoother the progression of the disease. Doctors believe this is due to the fact that younger people don't have the health issues to deal with that older patients have. Plus, their stronger, healthier bodies handle the difficulties much better. This is not always the case, but predominantly it works out as such.

The downside to being diagnosed at an early age is that Carbidopa/Levodopa typically isn't a viable option for them since the earlier you place a patient on it, the earlier the body begins to adjust to it, the effectiveness lessens and changes in medication have to be made to compensate for it down the road. Usually, young-onset patients are started on different medications that are also effective, leaving Carbidopa/Levodopa as a last resort for later on in their lives.

There is one other risk factor that contributes to your likelihood of developing Parkinson's: heavy metals (which we'll cover in greater detail in Chapter 13). Having a high concentration of these compounds in the body jacks up your risk considerably. And guess who had this issue?

Strike three.

Fact #3: Parkinson's disease is different from essential tremors.

There are considerably more Americans who suffer with essential tremors (ETs) than with Parkinson's (roughly 10 million compared to Parkinson's 1.5 million). While there is considerable on-going controversy as to whether or not essential tremors leads to Parkinson's, you have to consider that statistics show approximately 1 in 5 essential tremor patients do go on to develop Parkinson's. Also, some patients with essential tremors are at an increased risk of developing Parkinson's.

Essential tremors aren't largely talked about because they aren't considered to be as serious a condition as Parkinson's or other types of neurological disorders so the focus remains on the more serious conditions (not to say that ETs aren't serious). ETs also don't get much attention because there aren't any famous people who have them (the last one was the actress Katherine Hepburn). But it still doesn't hurt to know a little bit about them in case you know of someone who fits the description of symptoms.

The primary differences between Parkinson's and ETs are:

Parkinson's	ETs
Seen more during rest	Seen more during movement
Low intensity movements	High intensity movements
Wide range of symptoms	Tremors are primary symptom
Affects older people majority of the time	Range evenly involves all ages
Hands experience vast majority of tremors	Tremors often evenly affect hands, legs, head and Speech
Unaffected by alcohol	Improvement from alcohol
Starts on one side of body	Starts on both side simultaneously
Progression remains asymmetrical	Progresses

symmetrically/bilaterally

After the experiences I went through with being misdiagnosed, I would advise anyone who has been told that they have essential tremors to strongly consider talking to their doctor about the possibility of it being Parkinson's or the likelihood that it could develop into it later on. You need to know if it is, in fact, Parkinson's or a possibility that it could be one day so you can be placed on the right course of treatment as early on as possible.

Testosterone

Testosterone is classified as a steroid hormone that is found in large quantities in the testicles of men and in smaller amounts in the ovaries of women. Smaller amounts of it are also produced by the adrenal glands of both sexes.

Levels of testosterone in men are generally 7 to 8 times that of women with men producing approximately 20 times the amount of it on a daily basis as compared to what women produce, with the difference being utilized by different areas of the man's system. It is responsible for a wide range of functions from the growth of body hair to increasing bone and muscle mass and, of course, playing a critical role in sexual response.

A man's testosterone levels are at their highest when he is in his mid 30s. As men age, their level of testosterone begins to drop naturally at a rate of about 1 percent per year. But sometimes this drop can be excessive, usually caused by situations such as extreme and prolonged periods of stress or sudden and extreme life changes. When this happens, it ushers in symptoms ranging from fatigue and depression to the dreaded dropping of your libido.

What does low testosterone have to do with Parkinson's disease? Plenty.

Numerous studies have been conducted to determine if there was a connection between testosterone and Parkinson's. Not only did they find out what they wanted to know, but the extent of what they found out was absolutely shocking. It turns out that having low testosterone may very well be linked to the development of Parkinson's disease.

One of these studies, conducted by researchers at Rush University Medical Center in Chicago, and published in "The Journal of Biological Chemistry", showed that mice with low testosterone levels were developing Parkinson's disease. They also found that when older mice had low testosterone, there were fewer instances of Parkinson's.

What does this mean? In essence, it means that older mice had a higher level of protection from Parkinson's disease because of the presence of another important hormone: estrogen. As stated before, a man's testosterone drops as he ages, but at the same time, his estrogen levels begin to increase. Researchers believe that it is this increase in estrogen that helps to provide some protection from men contracting Parkinson's.

There is also some speculation that the reason why fewer women develop Parkinson's as compared to the number of men is due to women having a much higher level of estrogen. Mind you, this is all speculation and nothing has been proven, so far.

Where does this leave men? They have to be diligent.

If a younger man begins to notice a drop in their testosterone, they need to notify their doctor immediately. This doesn't mean that if their level begins to drop that they will develop Parkinson's disease, nor does it signify that their risk of Parkinson's automatically goes up. What it does mean is that having low testosterone may be linked to Parkinson's so it would be in their best interest to halt the decline as much as possible, as early on as possible.

For us older guys who have already been diagnosed with Parkinson's, we don't have to admit defeat-whether we have low testosterone or not. There is still plenty we can do about it.

Weight training is one of the best ways to increase your testosterone levels. Some other ways include:

- Increasing vitamin D
- Optimize your zinc levels
- Cut out sugar
- Eat healthy fats
- Reduce stress
- Lose weight

While you can take the easy way out and pop a pill if you need to beef up your testosterone, you're going to want to do it naturally. That's because testosterone creams and other man-made products have been under intense scrutiny by the FDA for causing a laundry list of medical conditions. In the end, it just isn't worth it to try to do it that way.

Chapter 3

Some Things I Learned About Parkinson's Disease

Did you know that there are different types of Parkinson's disease? I didn't know this going in. I assumed that it was a cookie-cutter type of disease and everyone with Parkinson's experienced the same effects, but that isn't the case- not by a long shot. It isn't the same thing as someone getting a cold and their symptoms are exactly like everyone else who has ever had a cold. Different kinds of Parkinson's means different types of treatments for different people involving different timetables and delivering different results.

The most common form of Parkinson's disease is idiopathic in nature, meaning it stems from an unknown cause. This type, also known as "tremor-dominant Parkinson's", affects 3 out of every 4 Parkinson patients, with symptoms typically beginning to surface while the patient is in their mid-forties to mid-fifties. It carries with it the usual symptoms of tremors, rigidity and slowing or freezing of movements, almost always starting in one hand and, over time, spreading to the opposite side of the body.

The second most common form of the disease is called "Partial Instability Gait Difficulty", or PIGD. This form of Parkinson's affects older individuals and is identifiable by a shuffling movement while walking, noticeable balance issues and frequent falls, all of which come on early in the disease. Since this form of Parkinson's has a faster progression than the tremor-dominant variety and since it does not respond well to standard Parkinson medications, including Levodopa, these patients face a harder road before them. People with PIGD often tend to develop dementia and cognitive difficulties quickly after developing Parkinson's.

There is also an atypical (or out of the ordinary) version known as Vascular Parkinson's. This type of Parkinson's disease occurs when a person experiences a reduction in blood flow to the brain, usually as a result of a stroke or possibly even another medical condition which targets circulation, such as diabetes. Symptoms closely resemble that of a stroke: slurred speech, difficulty swallowing or changing facial expression, difficulty concentrating and confusion. There can also be bowel issues such as incontinence.

Another form is known as Progressive Supranuclear Palsy, or PSP. Although it mimics many of the common symptoms of Parkinson's, there are a few differences. This form is more progressive than standard Parkinson's and almost all of these patients don't begin to experience symptoms until after age 50. Eventually, it leads to dementia. Currently, there are no treatment options available for PSP.

Corticobasal Degeneration is the least common variety of atypical Parkinson's and is characterized by rigidity and limb instability. The disease doesn't surface until after age 60 and, like PSP, progresses at a faster rate than Parkinson's. There are virtually no treatment options available and patients must rely on a clinical diagnosis for confirmation since there are no tests available that can be used to verify it.

A small percentage of the population experiences Drug-induced Parkinsonism. This is brought on by either taking amounts of a medication which are greater than usual or when these medications are taken for an extended period of time. The medications in question are those related to treating seizures or specific psychiatric disorders. The use of these medications doesn't exactly cause Parkinson's disease, but it does produce Parkinson-like symptoms. As the name implies, it is brought on by the use of certain prescription medications, which have the unfortunate side effect of lowering dopamine levels.

Lastly, the rarest form of the disease is Juvenile Parkinson's, affecting children and teenagers, which should not be confused with Early-Onset Parkinson's which tends to strike when the individual is in their twenties, thirties or forties. Patients who are in their forties when they are newly-diagnosed can also be referred to as Early-

Onset.

Being Misdiagnosed Is More Common Than You Might Think

In my case, I was first told that I had essential tremors. And I'm not an isolated case, either. In fact, people are misdiagnosed more often than you might think, not because the doctors are incompetent, but because early symptoms can be very misleading, leaving the doctors relatively little to go on.

If you present yourself to a doctor with mild symptoms, they don't have the luxury of being able to determine which direction your symptoms will go in the future. With that kind of limited information, they are forced to take a stab at what they anticipate for you and then prescribe medication accordingly. I have personally heard many cases where a doctor was stumped by the patient's symptoms and prescribed a Parkinson's medication with the intention being "if this helps, then we know it's Parkinson's. If it doesn't, then it's likely something else." It might sound like a radical or even an unorthodox approach, but sometimes that's all they have to work off of.

When you are in the early stages of Parkinson's disease, symptoms can be mild, making it rather difficult for a doctor to pinpoint exactly what the cause is. Of course, at the time, we don't know that we're dealing with Parkinson's so we aren't much help to them. Symptoms can be all over the board and can cause you to qualify for any number of different medical conditions so your doctor really doesn't have a whole lot to go on unless your symptoms are very pronounced. I admire them for taking on that kind of burden. I know *I* wouldn't want the responsibility of diagnosing what someone has.

Since there is no definitive test they can perform, they are pretty much left working off of their gut reaction, their training and their experience. But these can all become misleading if you happen to have symptoms that are less than textbook.

According to statistics gathered by the Michael J. Fox Foundation for Parkinson's Research, approximately 1 in 4 patients receive an initial misdiagnosis. What are some of the medical conditions that are often confused with Parkinson's?

- Benign essential tremors
- Multiple system atrophy
- Multiple sclerosis
- Amyotrophic lateral sclerosis (Lou Gehrig's disease)
- Supranuclear palsy
- Psuedobulbar palsy
- Huntington's disease
- Normal pressure hydrocephalus
- Wilson's disease
- Striato-nigral degeneration
- Hallervorden Spatz disease

Now that you see how much competition Parkinson symptoms have with being confused to other diseases, you can see why it's so important to get those additional opinions.

Diagnosing Parkinson's isn't an exact science so you have to be willing to be patient and understanding until your doctor can get things figured out. After all, they're learning and finding out things right along with you and there are constantly advancements in treatment and new research being conducted. I'll admit, there are some rare instances where a doctor can be incompetent or not aggressive enough with their treatment approach, but a vast majority of the time, they're doing the best that they can.

Fatigue

When you think of fatigue, you usually associate it with being overly tired due to work, illness, performing strenuous exercise, running your body down past it's limits or packing too much stress into your schedule. You can be physically fatigued, emotionally fatigued, mentally fatigued or sometimes even a combination of the three. But the truth is fatigue doesn't have to come from any of these sources. It can also come from your brain.

Dealing with fatigue is one thing, but dealing with fatigue when you have Parkinson's disease is something else, entirely. Parkinson patients with fatigue don't experience it because they're out of shape or because they try to pack too much into their day: it's because they can't help it. That's because unlike normal fatigue that only comes from tired muscles or stress, Parkinson's fatigue originates from a cellular level.

A common misconception is that fatigue means you need more sleep. But those with Parkinson's disease can be fatigued and not suffer from a loss of sleep because the fatigue isn't caused by it. Although insomnia and sleep interruptions can bring on fatigue, in these cases, they are not necessary for fatigue to exist. Also, a person who is sleepy will feel like taking a nap when the sleepiness hits them, whereas a person with Parkinson's can feel fatigued and still be wide awake.

While doctors aren't sure why people with Parkinson's disease have such a common occurrence of fatigue- and at such a high level- they do know that it isn't directly connected to a lack of sleep, cognitive decline or even the death of a high number of cells. And while medication can, and often does, have the side effect of causing fatigue, even this can't be held solely responsible for such a loss of energy, although timing of dosages can sometimes play a role in it if the patient isn't careful.

What they do know is that Parkinson sufferers have a much higher percentage of depression, partly due to the overwhelming presence of the fatigue. Ironically, patients who suffer from fatigue do so at the hands of depression, creating a vicious, unrelenting cycle. Parkinson fatigue can also be brought on due to trouble sleeping (for obvious reasons) and even pain from the muscles having to tense more as a coping mechanism to try to deal with the discomfort the body is feeling and/or from balance issues. Lastly, fatigue can come from a patient almost constantly fighting to gain control over involuntary movements and tremors.

But just because a Parkinson patient is overly fatigued doesn't mean that it necessarily has to do with Parkinson's. Sometimes, an individual can have other medical issues that are contributing to fatigue. Most often, these include type 2 diabetes, vitamin deficiencies and anemia.

A greater percentage of Parkinson sufferers have fatigue than not. And, to their dismay, fatigue is one of the earliest symptoms to appear. In fact, it often appears before a person is even diagnosed: they just don't yet know to put the two factors together. There is no rhyme or reason as to who will get fatigued and who won't. A young, newly-diagnosed Parkinson's patient can just as easily suffer from a greater degree of fatigue than someone who is older and has been diagnosed considerably longer.

There's also another critical problem with a Parkinson patient having fatigue and that is that it causes your symptoms to be more severe. Since being tired lowers your body's resistance to stress, this allows stress to attack you with a greater intensity, directly worsening your symptoms, which is why rest is so important.

Another common issue is that someone with Parkinson's can feel more energized one day than the next without changing their routine. Getting the same amount of sleep, eating virtually the same meals and performing the same tasks has no bearing on how much energy they will experience from day-to-day. This makes it virtually impossible to know how fatigued you'll be on a regular basis and even more difficult to plan ahead.

Fatigue is particularly damaging to a Parkinson patient because by zapping your energy, you are less likely to want to exercise. Since exercise plays such a pivotal role in Parkinson therapy, cutting back on exercise is not a good plan and can have a devastating effect on the progression of the disease, placing an even heavier burden on the individual. After all, if a patient is constantly fatigued they don't feel like exercising. But not exercising means that your muscles become weaker, lowering your energy levels and turning the entire situation into a dangerous downward spiral- not to mention dramatically upping your risk of becoming depressed.

So what can be done about fatigue? While a simple approach would be to try to overpower it with different medication, this isn't a practical answer because you're dealing with more than just someone who is overwhelmed with life circumstances. You're also dealing with someone who is suffering from lots and lots of stress. Plus, if you choose to go the route of additional medication you usually only end up making matters worse because the medication has its own side effects that you now have to contend with, which just creates more problems and, sadly, makes you more fatigued mentally. But that doesn't mean all hope is lost. Since fatigue is so closely related to stress, I'm going to share a secret with you in Chapter 10 that's going to do wonders for dealing with both.

Arm Movements

Roughly 70 percent of Parkinson patients will notice an abnormal tremor in one foot or hand as an early sign of the disease. Eventually, the tremor will spread bilaterally to both sides. The tremor can be described as either an oscillating or a shaking movement and occurs tends to occur when the individual is at rest. When they begin to move the affected extremity, the shaking stops. Since the tremors are associated with the muscles while they are not at work, this is referred to as "resting tremors" and is a classic early symptom of Parkinson's.

Abnormal arm movements can also be detected while an individual is walking. This is seen as the individual not swinging one of their arms as freely as the other, making it appear more rigid. Although both arms can eventually shake or be limited in movement, the shaking or erratic arm swinging will always be more apparent in the arm initially affected.

Skin Problems

Your skin is the largest organ of your body; yet, few realize that even this area is not spared from the effects of Parkinson's disease.

There are a few telltale symptoms of the skin that are an unfortunate part of having Parkinson's. It doesn't mean that everyone will have all of these symptoms, but the likelihood that some or all of these will occur in patients does increase with each advancing stage of the disease.

1. Seborrhea. These are greasy skin areas, most typically on the forehead and around the nose. Scientists are not sure why Parkinson targets these particular areas of skin, but they do know that it has something to do with the dramatic drop in dopamine levels in the skin glands.

2. Dermatitis. Sometimes, seborrhea can be a pre-cursor to dermatitis. When this occurs, it is usually not due to a lack of cleanliness, but due to Parkinson's, itself. Studies have shown that when dopamine leaves are elevated, such as when medicaments are administered, the dermatitis coincidentally begins to improve.

It has been shown that having inaccurate levels of dopamine- either too much or too little- can exacerbate excessive sweating, or hyperhidrosis. For example, if someone with Parkinson's begins to experience excessive sweating during "off" times, upping their dosage of dopamine tends to remedy the problem. Of course, this issue should be discussed with your doctor before any adjustments to medications are made. Parkinson patients who suffer from hyperhidrosis tend to sweat more around the head and neck only. The most common time this occurs is during sleep, causing the individual to wake up with a sweat-soaked pillow while the rest of the body stays relatively dry.

There have been some concerns about a higher prevalence of skin lesions, both cancerous and non-cancerous, in Parkinson patients. While studies are still ongoing, no direct connection has been made for Parkinson's patients being at a higher risk of developing skin lesions. However, there is reason for concern for Parkinson patients who also suffer with malignant melanomas. Although further studies are still being made to make the connection between Parkinson's disease and malignant melanomas, the theory is that both melanin and dopamine may actually use the same biochemical trails throughout the body.

Stages of Parkinson's

Parkinson's disease can be broken down into five distinct stages. After an office evaluation, your doctor will be able to classify which stage they feel you have entered into based on either the Hoehn or Yahr rating system, or the Unified Parkinson's Disease Rating Scale. Since Parkinson's is such a silent and hidden disease, an individual can easily have entered the second or even third stage of Parkinson's before making a connection between the symptoms they are experiencing and the disease.

While the Hoehn and Yahr rating systems focus primarily on classic Parkinson's symptoms such as tremors and rigidity, the Unified Parkinson's Disease Rating Scale is preferred by some doctors because it also takes into account other key issues such as task impairment and cognitive difficulties.
This gives them a broader expanse of issues with which to make an assessment.

Doctors rely on the presence and/or severity of primary Parkinson symptoms to determine how advanced the disease has become. Noting these symptoms gives the doctor a good determination as to which stage the patient has progressed to. The symptoms used for this assessment are:

- tremors
- stiffness of extremities
- bradykinesia, or slowing of movements
- balance or walking issues

During a routine office visit, your doctor uses different movement exercises to determine how far your symptoms have progressed. Some of the movement shuteye will ask you to perform might seem a little ridiculous, but to your doctor, it provides volumes of information.

The Five Stages of Parkinson's disease

Unfortunately, there is no accurate way to determine how long someone will remain in each stage. The best that we can hope for is to slow down the progression as much as possible through lifestyle choices. Here are the five stages:

Stage 1: Unilateral tremors. These may be so minute that, in some instances, they may be practically invisible. Since they typically only occur on one side of the body in the beginning, they are often dismissed without concern. The fact that they are generally so mild means that they do not disrupt the individual's lifestyle.

Stage 2: Symptoms spread bilaterally. By now, symptoms have progressed to the point that the individual begins to notice them and they are beginning to interfere with their everyday activities. This is usually the point at which the individual sees a specialist and receives a diagnosis. Besides tremors, the individual will typically see a noticeable difference in their facial expressions, changes in the volume of their voice, they may possibly begin to have balance issues and maybe even some rigidity. The progression from stage one to stage two could range from only a few months to several years, or possibly even longer, depending on how proactive the individual becomes with exercise and disease management.

Stage 3: Overall symptoms worsen. Symptoms of stage two and stage three are quite similar except for the fact that with stage 3 there is a noticeable difficulty with balance and gait. This dramatically increases the likelihood of falls occurring. For this reason, entering stage three is considered to be a major turning point in the progression of the disease. Despite the increased hindrances, the individual is usually still able to remain independent.

Stage 4: Patient loses some independence. By this stage, symptoms have progressed to the point that the patient requires assistance to get around. Balance and gait are a definite issue, resulting in either the use of a can or walker or the assistance of another individual. These individuals may still be able to live on their own, but it is something that requires careful consideration because of the increased fear of falls.

Stage 5: Total assistance required. These patients are unable to stand and require the use of a wheelchair due to advanced freezing and increased rigidity of the legs. Also, there is usually a presence of confusion, delusions and hallucinations. At this point, the benefits of medications are overshadowed by the side effects they bring, thus, these individual oftentimes discontinue medication since it is no longer serving a purpose, leaving these individual in need of round-the-clock care.

Chapter 4

More Common Symptoms of Parkinson's Disease That You Might Initially Overlook

Besides the characteristic symptom of tremors, there are other undeniable signs that help to define Parkinson's disease for what it is. But that doesn't mean that everyone with this disease will have the same exact set of symptoms. The fact is, different people can have different symptoms surfacing at different times. Along with how closely Parkinson's mirrors essential tremors, it often makes it difficult for doctors to diagnose between the two in the early stages of the disease. This is what happened to me.

Here are a few primary symptoms of Parkinson's that you may, or may not, already have:

1. Bradykinesia. This refers to the slowing of movements. It might be one of the symptoms typically associated with Parkinson's, but bradykinesia isn't just restricted to this one disease. Bradykinesia can also be found in other forms of neurological disorders, too.

The two most common symptoms of bradykinesia are tremors and rigidity. But, ironically, Parkinson treatment is not geared towards treating the tremors or the rigidity, as most people erroneously believe, but rather on the bradykinesia, itself. The tremors and the rigidity are merely symptoms of the bradykinesia, and *not* the actual cause. These tremors are referred to as "resting tremors" because they don't require exertion for them to occur. In fact, they typically go away once the affected extremely is put into motion. Having bradykinesia affects the quality of a Parkinson patient's much more than either the tremors or the rigidity does.

Many classic Parkinson symptoms fall under the umbrella category of bradykinesia. These include arm swinging, a slower walking pace, loss or decrease in facial expression, smaller handwriting, lower tone of voice, having difficulty swallowing, slower movement sand having difficulty rolling over in bed.

2. Cogwheel rigidity. This refers to your movements not being fluid, but rather "robotic" in appearance. Instead of an easy flow to your movements, such as moving your arm to pick something up, there are sharp, temporary pauses in the movement. The reason it is called cogwheel rigidity is because it resembles the ratcheted movements of a cogwheel, such as you would find in a clock.

3. Joint pain. Joint pain classification is based on the level of separation between the pain receptors of the tissue and the nerves that are responsible for transmitting the pain signals. The three categories are:

- neuropathic- the pain originates from the nerves, themselves
- nociceptive- the pain originates from the nerves, skin and the tissue surrounding them, which means there is actual tissue damage
  or
- a combination of both

The majority of pain that individuals with Parkinson's experience is nociceptive pain. This means that the tissue surrounding the nerve receptors have either already become injured or has the potential of being injured. The injury can be due to any number of things from inflammation to a fall.

One common area for a Parkinson's patient to have joint pain is in the shoulder (not necessarily the dominant shoulder). This is often mistaken as being a condition known as "frozen shoulder" and can present itself years before other symptoms come about. I was diagnosed with frozen shoulder some four years before I was diagnosed with Parkinson's.

4 Dyskinesia. These are involuntary movements, sometimes referred to as "tics", where parts of the body, typically the arms, begin to move rhythmically on their own. Dyskinesia occurs because of one of two reasons:

- because of a reaction to stress
- prolonged use of Levodopa or certain antipsychotic medications

Actor Michael J. Fox is a prime example of someone with dyskinesia. Many think that the repetitive, jerking movements that they see are from the Parkinson's, when, in fact, it's mostly a side effect of his medications. Also, the more stress a Parkinson's patient is under, the more pronounced the dyskinesia will appear. This is another reason why reducing the stress in your life is vital. Those who have been on Levodopa for an extended period of time will also likely see dyskinesia begin to surface as time progresses. Dyskinesia usually doesn't occur in the early stages of Parkinson's, but is reserved for later stages.

It's a common misconception by some that dyskinesia is usually brought on due to the side effects of Parkinson medications. Others believe that it is a product of the disease itself, coming on automatically as time, and the intensity of the disease, progresses. But the truth is that neither of these, alone, are the case. Dyskinesia tends to occur because of a combination of the side effects of Parkinson medications *and* a prolonged duration of the disease. Unfortunately, there is no effective treatment for dyskinesia except to stifle stress as much as possible.

5. Olfactory dysfunction. At some point, loss of olfaction, or sense of smell, affects over 95 percent of Parkinson's patients, making it a critical diagnosing tool and another way to track a patient's progression of the disease. In comparison, the percentage of individuals over the age of 55 who do not have Parkinson's and experience some form of olfactory dysfunction is only around 25 percent. Most Parkinson's patients report that a loss of olfactory senses was noticed a few years prior to them starting to experience a decline in their motor skills.

The sad part concerning a loss of olfaction is the impact it has on eating since flavor is derived from both smelling *and* tasting. Alone, the human tongue is only capable of registering four types of flavor: salty, bitter, sweet and sour, which means that everything else is registered by our sense of smell. When our sense of smell diminishes, we lose the ability to distinguish a complexity of flavors and have to rely on just the four basic ones that the tongue registers. In other words, we rely heavily on our sense of smell to help us anticipate what we are about to enjoy.

6. Blank/stiff facial expression. This symptom, known as "facial masking", refers to the facial muscles becoming immobile. To the casual observer, Parkinson's patients with facial masking appear to be bored or uninterested in the topic being discussed, but, in actuality, someone with Parkinson's doesn't even realize that their face is void of expression.

The face is made up of approximately 45 muscles that generate every expression from frowning to smiling. Since the large majority of communication comes from our face, not having a normal range of expressions can come across in a negative manner to others.

7. Dystonia. This third most common type of movement disorder isn't just confined to Parkinson's patients: even children can develop it. It is characterized by prolonged periods of twisting and involuntary muscle contractions, which result in pain and can affect your posture, as well as your movements. Dystonia typically begins in one isolated body apart and then spreads to others. Affected areas include the face, vocal cords, neck, shoulders, back, arms and legs.

Although dystonia can occur in many parts of the body, believe it or not the most common area that a Parkinson patient will experience dystonia is in the big toe. The condition causes it to point slightly upward while the remainder of the toes continue to stay straight. Even though it can be painful and make normal movements difficult, most people with dystonia are able to lead a relatively normal life. It is only in extreme cases where the patient will require medical assistance. Flare-ups of dystonia are worse first thing in the morning or when the individual is under increased amounts of stress.

Although the origin of dystonia comes from the same region of the brain affected by Parkinson's, the basal ganglia, the cause of the disease is still unknown. Like Parkinson's, dystonia could be caused by adverse environmental conditions or even genetics. The treatment for dystonia is medications and, in extreme cases, deep brain stimulation (DBS), which we'll cover later. Physical therapy or types of movement practices, such as yoga, Pilates and Tai chi are also beneficial.

8. Weakened voice. Since Parkinson's affects the strength and control of muscles, it stands to reason that the disease will eventually affect a patient's voice. There is no actual damage to the muscles themselves, but rather a reduction of airflow, as well as a reduction in the throat's effort to speak in a normal fashion. This also makes it difficult for the individual to swallow.

As Parkinson's worsens, the muscles of the voice box often begin to lose their control, strength and coordination, which, in turn, will affect the individual's speech. Besides the obvious sign of a loss in volume, telltale signs of a weakened voice include a monotone quality (void of expression), pauses before speech can be initiated, a slurring of speech, short pauses between words and even a tremulous voice, such as the one experienced by the actress Katherine Hepburn. The only real treatment for a weakened voice is voice therapy.

9. Dysphagia. Dysphagia, or difficulty swallowing, is caused by uncoordinated movements of the muscles in the mouth and throat and affects as many as 8 out of every 10 Parkinson patients at some point.

10. Balance issues. This is a major issue for those with Parkinson's since injuries sustained from a fall due to a loss of balance are one of the primary causes of death in these patients. The best way to ward off this symptom is do strengthen your core, legs and back.

Balance issues can also include retropulsion, or the sensation of falling backwards. This is why a neurologist will stand behind you and pull back on your shoulders to check for postural stability as par of their evaluation. This tells them the likelihood of you experiencing a fall by losing your balance going backwards.

11. Stooped posture. Identifying this as being a sign of Parkinson's can be a bit tricky since it is the usual inclination for many individuals to stoop forward as they advance in years. But while it might be common for this type of postural change to affect older people, Parkinson's disease manages to accelerate this condition.

Since Parkinson's brings about rigidity, or a change to muscle tone, this rigidity interferes with the normal flexibility of the muscle fibers and instead of allowing them a full, normal range of motion, holds them tightly in place. As a result, these muscle fibers begin to shorten, making it even more difficult for them to allow movement.

By not allowing the muscles to extend to their full capacity, the posture begins to pull forward. Sometimes, instead of pulling forward, an individual will pull to one side. In either case, this contributes a great deal to a loss of balance and episodes of falls because the head, which is the center of mass for the body and where your equilibrium originates, is thrown off. Being unnaturally pulled forward or to the side can also interfere with normal breathing, making it shallow and labored.

Having a stooped posture also brings about another concern: unwanted accelerations when walking. Since the tendency of the Parkinson-ridden body is to stoop forward, this throws off the body's center of gravity. Since their body is now slanted forward, the body's normal reaction is to lean in that direction as the individual begins to take steps, creating an unnecessary and somewhat accelerated momentum. The individual can easily find themselves taking steps too quickly, lose their balance and fall.

12. Chronic constipation. Constipation strikes people with Parkinson's more than the average individual because of how the disease attacks the autonomic nervous system, which is the part of the nervous system that controls those bodily functions that are automatic and not consciously directed (heart beats, breathing,etc.) Since Parkinson's disease disrupts the autonomic system, it disrupts normal, smooth muscle moments, such as, in this case, bowl movements.

13. Urinary urgency (also known as urinary dysfunction).
Parkinson patients soon realize that their condition doesn't just cause disruptions in movements, but that it also creates certain "non motor" symptoms that affect the autonomic parts of the nervous system. The term autonomic means "automatic", or functions in the body that can be referred to as being on "autopilot". These functions include everything from the beating of your heart all the way down to urination.

Urinary issues are common for Parkinson sufferers. They include frequent urination which causes the individual to have to go more than a typical number of times during the day, even though the bladder might not be full or close to full, a disruption of sleep (known as nocturia) and urinary urgency. Other common problems include a condition known as hesitancy, meaning the individual has to push in order to empty their bladder and having a weaker stream of urine even though the sensation to urinate may seem high. The last, and most common issue, urinary urgency means the bladder senses that it needs emptying and the individual is unable to postpone doing so once the body perceives this sensation.

14. Drooling. Also known as "dribbling", or by the medical term "sialorrhoea", this is another unfortunate and embarrassing symptom that occurs in most Parkinson patients- especially as their disease progresses.

Despite popular belief, drooling is not caused by an increase in saliva. Rather, it is due to a decrease in the natural tendency to swallow. Add this to a "frozen" expression, a tendency for the mouth to slightly hang open, the head to be slightly tilted forward due to having a stooped frame and a decreased awareness and this combination culminates into drooling.

In order to alleviate this problem, some doctors may try to prescribe anti-cholinergics, which are intended to dry out the mouth and, thus, reduce the amount of saliva that collects. But these are not always a practical approach, especially for older patients as they come with their own set of side effects. Possible side effects include blurred vision, drowsiness, excitement, hallucinations, behavioral issues and even interference with urinary issues. The safest approach would be to have the individual see a Speech and Language therapist who can train them on working to better control their ability to swallow.

15. Osteoporosis. Individuals with Parkinson's are not only at an increased risk of osteoporosis (brittle or fragile bones), but also for osteopenia (thinning bones). Many studies have been conducted on both conditions and there is a clear and undeniable connection between both types of bone disintegration and Parkinson's disease. Scientists believe that such a strong connection is caused by the disruption of signals to the bones from Parkinson's, causing the bones to become thin and brittle. Since Parkinson's patients are at such an increased risk for falls, osteoporosis and osteopenia are major concerns that should always be immediately addressed.

Regular bone health and density examinations by your doctor are a necessity. The best recourse to help ward off these conditions is to get plenty of vitamin D, supplement with calcium (if your calcium intake is less-than-favorable) and exercise.

16. Smaller handwriting. It's called "micrographia" and it eventually afflicts every Parkinson patient.
The truth of the matter is that most people don't notice a change in their handwriting becoming smaller until it is pointed out to them by someone else- often their neurologist. But this is such a classic symptom that it is one of the first tests given by your doctor when they begin to suspect that a patient might have Parkinson's.

17. Hypnic jerk. The shortened name of "hypnagogic jerk" and also known as "sleep twitch", "night start" or "sleep start", this is a sudden, involuntary jolting movement of the body which occurs just as you are falling asleep. The severity of the jolting movement often awakens you. The sensation resembles what you experience when you are suddenly frightened and is typically followed by a sensation that you are falling.

18. Stiffness. Instead of having a smooth, fluid movement of their extremities, a Parkinson patient will have stiffness. The range of motion may be limited or the range may be there, but the ease with which the extremities move has been noticeably reduced.

The Problem of Freezing

Also known as "motor block", freezing refers to both an inability to start a motion and an inability to stop a repetitive or rhythmic motion once it has been generated. The cause of freezing in Parkinson's is unknown.

Doctors are not able to explain exactly why some Parkinson patients are more susceptible to freezing than others, but experience does show us that the likelihood of experiencing a freezing episode increases as a patient's disease progresses. Freezing is also quite common when a Parkinson patient's medications begin to wear off, known as their "off" time. It's like turning off a light switch because one second you're moving and then, suddenly, you aren't. It's happens just that quick and then, after a brief pause, your normal movements return just as quickly as they were shut off. The only problem is that you never know *when* it's going to happen.

The most common example of freezing involves repetitive movement of the hands, such as when you're brushing your teeth, but other ways that freezing can affect you is while you're writing, walking, talking or even doing something as basic as blinking.

Freezing that occurs when an individual is walking and has to make a decision, such as turning a corner or entering a room, is referred to as "gait hesitation". This also places the individual at an increased risk of tripping and falling. Why would something as simple as entering a doorway interfere with walking? Because it takes the brain's focus off of walking and focuses it on the doorway and where you will go once you pass through it. The solution to this dilemma is to force yourself to focus your attention away from the doorway and back to your walking.

When a Parkinson's patient is walking with someone, they can sometimes find the individual's presence a distraction, which can subsequently lead to freezing of their gait. This is due to the problem Parkinson patents can have with multi-tasking. The best way to avoid this is to politely ask the individual accompanying you not to talk to you while you are trying to walk so that your attention is not diverted.

Becoming frozen strikes out of nowhere and can occur at any time without any warning. For example, if an individual becomes frozen while walking, they will be temporarily unable to move their feet, as if they are cemented in place. This is why being at an increased risk of falling is a major concern for Parkinson patents since both the start and the end of a freezing episode cannot be predicted with any form of accuracy, catching the individual completely off-guard. Other common examples of when freezing occurs is when you're tying your shoes or shampooing your hair. Anything that involves a rhythmic motion is an opportunity for your body to freeze.

Episodes of freezing usually only last for 5 to 10 seconds. Once your brain "resets" itself, the movements can continue once again. These episodes are not isolated incidences, either. A patient can experience several freezing episodes while trying to complete a single task. Besides being a nuisance, freezing can also cause an individual to fall due to their feet stopping their forward movement abruptly.

What are the some things to do when you encounter a freezing episode? The best thing to do is to break the brain's sequence of the event by distraction and one of the best ways to accomplish this is by singing. Other successful methods include stepping over an "imaginary" line on the floor, using a laser pointer to pinpoint a "target" on the floor out in front of you that you can proceed towards, taking a single step sideways and then restarting the walking, shifting the weight to the other foot or even playing some rhythmic music to distract you. As you can see, the prevailing point is to distract the brain so it can redirect it's focus off of the freezing and back on to movement.

If a caregiver is present during a freezing episode, have the caregiver stand off to the individual's side and place one of their own feet horizontally in front of the patient's feet and then ask them to take a step over it. This movement will typically break the freezing cycle and allow them to continue walking.

Another good way to avoid gait hesitation is to avoid pivoting when walking. Pivoting is common in Parkinson patients when they are required to make a turn. Instead of switching directions in a fluid motion, the Parkinson patient will pivot in one position until they are facing their desired direction. The way around this is to make a wider swing of movements, taking several additional steps outward, creating a wider circle instead of trying to make a sharper turn.

Some of these symptoms of Parkinson's are seen early-on in the disease while others have to slowly develop over time- sometimes not surfacing for many years. There's no concrete way of determining which symptoms will appear in what order and how much time will elapse between each one or even if an individual will experience them at all. That brings us to the next thing I wish I'd known when first diagnosed:

Insight #3: Everybody progresses at different rates.

Trying to determine exactly how Parkinson's disease will affect your life and how quickly it will do so is not an exact science. It would be great if there were a cookie-cutter rate of progression that you could rely on where you could anticipate exactly which symptoms you were going to develop, when you would develop them and how severe they would become, in order for you to sufficiently plan ahead accordingly, but that's just simply not the case.

The fact is some Parkinson patients will progress at a much faster rate than others. This doesn't always have to do with the individual, but has more to do with how genetics and the type and severity of their Parkinson's comes into play here. There is only so much control you have before genetics takes over. But make no mistake about it: you *do* have quite a bit of control.

Some will experience a higher level of relief from specific medications than others. Some won't react at all from certain meds.

Some will need more meds to stabilize the effects while others will manage with minimal assistance from prescriptions. It's virtually impossible to tell in advance how someone's way of life will be negatively impacted by the disease or the side effects they will experience from medication since it's set strictly on an individual basis. The only thing that your doctor can do to help is to keep a close eye on the improvement or worsening of your symptoms to tell you what changes need to be made accordingly.

Your rate of progression depends on a number of factors:

- your current level of health
- your weight
- the frequency and intensity of your exercise program
- your medications
- your diet

As I mentioned earlier, most patients may have already advanced into the second or sometimes even the third stage of Parkinson's by the time they reach a diagnosis. This doesn't mean you're too late to do anything about it so don't ever let your mind go there. It *does* mean that you need to be proactive about your treatment because the clock is ticking…ticking…ticking… With Parkinson's disease, it's always ticking.

The unsettling truth is that you can remain in a particular stage of Parkinson's for years- in some instances, even a decade or more. There's no way of telling exactly how long you will remain in a particular stage because, again, everyone is different, every situation is different and everyone responds differently to medications. The rate at which you progress also has a lot to do with your lifestyle and how much of a stand you take with it. It's like buying a luxury car. If you do the proper types of maintenance on it and take care of it and protect it, it will perform much better and last you longer than if you neglect it and take it for granted.

You might not be able to determine your rate of progression, but there are two things that you can be sure of: (1) your current set of symptoms will gradually become worse as time goes on, and (2) over time, you will develop new symptoms. That isn't meant to depress you or in any way take away your hope. As brutal as that truth may sound, it doesn't means that the course of your life is set in stone. It's a realization that you have to be willing to accept so you know what you're going to be up against. It also tells you things to be on the lookout for that you might not otherwise make the connection to Parkinson's.

Sadly, upon hearing the news of having Parkinson's, many choose to accept it as a death sentence and they sit idly by awaiting the inevitable. But the inevitable is *not* what you perceive it to be. Even though Parkinson's disease will do its best to determine the quality of your life, you can take consolation in knowing that it will not necessarily shorten your life.

Yes, Parkinson's is a degenerative disease so it will get worse as time goes on. But it does not call ALL the shots. It might set the stage for the introduction of other types of complications that can arise from it, but, again, this is not completely set in stone. It also doesn't determine exactly how quickly it will progress. YOU have a great deal of input in the rate of your disease's progression. If you just sit around doing nothing, feeling sorry for yourself and waiting for the inevitable time when the disease completely takes over your life, then you will lose out on living and life itself. But if you take a stand and decide not to allow *it* to run your life, but for *you* to run it, then you will live, instead of just existing. You have to take a proactive approach or Parkinson's will win.

Chapter 5

How Parkinson's Disease Affects Your Family

Like any illness, it's impossible for a Parkinson's sufferer to fully explain what they're going through to their spouse and family. Your family can see that you're experiencing issues and they even see your daily struggles, but despite all of that sympathy and understanding it's still difficult to put yourself in someone else's illness. That doesn't mean that the spouses and family don't understand the dilemma within reason because they're close enough to you that they can see when you're hurting emotionally. They see your struggles, your limitations, your frustrations and your challenges. And although they aren't physically occupying your body, they do understand what's happening so it's important that you know how much it hurts them to see what you're going through with this disease.

Standing by and watching someone you love and care for gradually lose some of the quality of their life through the years is sheer torture. What makes it even worse is knowing that there's nothing you can do to take away the disease. Sure, you can improve their lives by being there for them, but it still feels hopeless to know that there's no cure. Even if a loved one is able to assist the patient in their everyday life, at least to an extent, they still feel helpless because there is only so much they can do for them.

There is such a wide range of emotions that you go through when first diagnosed, you really need to have the support of your family and friends behind you so you don't feel as if you have to try to go through it alone. If you have someone available who can help you get through it, it takes a lot of pressure off of the Parkinson patient so they can focus more on their health, which is exactly what needs to happen. They're still going to be concerned, but if it takes even a small measure of the burden from their shoulders, it's well worth it.

Having someone to be an advocate on your behalf- especially at doctor appointments- is crucial. There is such a wealth of knowledge and instruction being shared during an office visit that it's very easy to overlook or completely miss out on something that could adversely affect the patient's health and well-being. Parkinson patients- particularly those who are newly-diagnosed- need to be able to concentrate more on what their doctor is saying to them without being so fixated on their emotional state. In the beginning, this flood of new information is overwhelming, to say the least. They're still trying to come to grips with what's going on while so much is being thrown at them all at once so the possibility that they might miss hearing an important detail goes up dramatically.

Anytime a Parkinson patient goes to the doctor, it's a blatant reminder of what they're going through so it's not always easy to take in all of the information being shared- especially when changes are being made, such as to medications, for example. Having an advocate available at your appointments not only reduces the risk of missing out on key pieces of information, but just the moral support alone that it provides the patient is priceless.

But all of the responsibility doesn't fall on their immediate family. Parkinson patients also need to be understanding towards their friends and extended family. As a patient, we're going to have good days and, unfortunately, we're going to have some bad days. We just have to remember that our family is there for us- no matter what- and we can't take our frustration or impatience out on them. We might not feel good, but we can't let the disease win. We need to remember how invaluable their support is to us.

As far as friends go, you're going to see a wide range of reactions when they first find out about your condition. You can never control how people react to your diagnosis so don't worry about trying to do so. What you can do is try to put them at ease as much as possible by showing them that you've accepted it and that they should, too. If you act like it's just a hurdle that you're going to have to deal with and it's nothing you aren't willing to fight for then it takes some of the burden off of them. They'll want to be there for you, but they won't know how. You have to remember that this is all new to them, as well.

Probably the biggest concern that your friends will have is whether or not to be sad for you. Human nature tends to say that they will be, but they will also be unsure if they should convey that sadness to you because on one hand, they'll want to let you know that they sympathize with you, but on the other hand, they don't want to let you see that they're worried because they don't want to cause you any unnecessary worry. You have to understand that it's a delicate line that they're standing on- especially if it's the first time they've ever been placed in that position. They're venturing into new territory just as much as you.

If you want to help them help you, and since knowledge is power, the best thing you can do for everyone involved is help them to understand what Parkinson's disease is so they'll know what to expect. Knowing ahead of time what to expect will not only allow them to help you deal with what you're going through, but the more you talk about it, the more comfortable you'll become with it.

Friends should never try to treat you differently just because you have Parkinson's. They might think that they're protecting you while, in actuality, they're refusing to face reality. They may have your best interests at heart, but ignoring the situation is only going to succeed in doing more harm than good. If they try to go this route, show them that you're the same person you've always been. The bottom line is that they need to focus on your abilities- not your limitations. They can feel compassion without sympathy. They can offer help instead of pity. How they react to you helps to determine how you react to them and your total outlook.

But understand that as your disease progresses, it's going to put more and more of a strain on your relationships. Friends, particularly, may feel uncomfortable around you simply because they don't know how to handle it. That's just natural. You have to be willing to communicate openly with your family, friends, coworkers and especially with your spouse. They need to know what you're feeling so when you are having a not-so-good day, they'll know the reason behind it and help you to move past it. We all need help getting through this. It isn't any fun, but it's even less fun when we don't have the support of others behind us.

We have to remain as optimistic as possible as we go down this difficult and challenging road. It will only feel like the end of the world if we let it.

Chapter 6

How Parkinson's Disease Affects You Mentally

Although most of the information you read about Parkinson's disease tends to focus on the physical changes that you will experience, there are also other areas of a patient's life that are radically affected. Since Parkinson's is a disease that targets the brain, it stands to reason that it can cause other types of symptoms that are more emotional in nature than just the standard physical ones that we are accustomed to dealing with. But these changes don't just cause a shift in your emotions. Some of them radically and adversely affect the disease, itself. If the person isn't willing to deal with these issues as soon as they present themselves, they risk bringing unnecessary complications into the picture, giving the disease even more control over their life. Emotional changes need to be addressed as much as the physical ones since choosing to ignore them isn't going to make them go away.

The emotional side of Parkinson's is just as important as the physical side, making the two strongly connected. As a Parkinson's patient begins to fixate more and more on the decline of their health- even if the rate of decline is gradual and not really noticeable- it can have a huge impact on how they perceive life, in general. It can also cause them to lose hope and begin to concede to the disease, forgoing exercise and other important lifestyle changes that can help to prolong and improve the quality of their life. As soon as an individual starts to care less about their situation, the progression of their disease will automatically begin to accelerate and, as a result, their overall health will decline. This is why maintaining a healthy emotional state is vital to the management of Parkinson's.

One major problem with Parkinson's is that the hippocampus portion of the brain, which is the control center for your emotions, becomes damaged by the effects of the disease and, subsequently, begins to shrink. The loss of this brain tissue correlates with a lowered emotional state, making depression and other psychiatric conditions more likely to occur.

It is imperative that those with Parkinson's remain always optimistic since remaining positive goes a long way in helping you make good decisions that will keep the disease at bay as much as possible. But I'm not going to lie to you and say that it won't be challenging at times. Given how Parkinson's directly affects the chemicals in your brain, remaining optimistic can be rather difficult, to say the least.

Depression

It has been said that the difference between anxiety and depression can be summed up in a simple comparison:

> anxiety means you care *too* much about *everything*;
> depression means you *don't* care about *anything*.

With the radical fluctuation of brain chemicals that takes place it's no wonder that Parkinson's disease increases the likelihood that you'll suffer from some level of depression. Studies show that up to 60 percent of Parkinson patients see at least a mild to moderate increase in depressive symptoms, with the occurrence increasing as symptoms increase and the patient's quality of life becomes more and more affected. But there's a very good reason why there is such a strong connection between these depression and Parkinson's.

We know that Parkinson's disease affects several parts of the brain that have to do with your emotions. While one of these areas, the frontal lobe, works to regulate your mood, the downside is that it also allows you to fixate on negative events in your life. Since Parkinson's disease damages the frontal lobe, becoming obsessed with these dark periods becomes much easier.

Sadly, damage to the frontal lobe is what happened to the actor, Robin Williams, whom we just lost in August of 2014. He had just been diagnosed with Parkinson's, but had become completely overwhelmed with the depression that accompanied it. The combination of his depression and the darkness that his new diagnosis finally became too much for him to handle and he took his own life. A year later, his family discovered that Williams had also suffered from dementia with Lewy bodies (DLB), a rapidly progressing and unrelenting condition that accelerated the deterioration of William's health and outlook.

DLB hadn't received a lot of attention in the past until Williams was diagnosed with it shortly before his death, even though it is ranked as the second most common cause of dementia in older individuals, ranked behind Alzheimer's disease.

DLB occurs when globs of the protein alpha-synuclein begin to accumulate within the brain's nerve cells for reasons which still remind a mystery to researchers. Although these clumps of destructive protein can be found in various regions of the brain, it is when they become concentrated within the substantia nigra that dopamine levels become depleted, forming Parkinson's.

But as damaging a single episode of depression can be it can also be crippling because of it's higher rate of recurrence. If an individual, even someone without Parkinson's, suffers from clinical depression, is able to resolve their issues, their chances of once again becoming clinically depressed are increased by more than 15 percent. In other words, the more often your brain succumbs to the effects of depression, the more likely you are to repeat that pattern again down the road. Throw Parkinson's disease into the mix and you're really setting yourself up for a challenge.

Research shows that certain psychiatric conditions, namely depression, tends to surface years before the individual begins to experience a change in their motor skills or physical abilities. Even though the psychiatric change can take place as much as a decade before common Parkinson symptoms are realized, many patients fail to make the connection between the two until after they are diagnosed with Parkinson's and learn how much of an influence Parkinson's can have on depression.

Diagnosing depression in Parkinson's patients can be challenging simply because both conditions share so many common symptoms, such as:

- weight loss
- trouble sleeping
- lower libido
- a feeling of uncaring
- feeling pessimistic
- being irritable or impatient
- a loss of interest in usual activities
- socially reserved
- sleeping far too much or too often
- fatigue
- difficulty with concentration and decision making
- significant drop in mood
- feeling worthless or guilty for no apparent reason
- having dark thoughts

The best way to distinguish between the symptoms that can be directly tied to Parkinson's and those which are a result of depression is that symptoms of depression tend to come on quicker than those of Parkinson's. With depression, an outsider can see a noticeable difference in an individual's demeanor in as little as a few days to no more than a few weeks, whereas symptoms tied to Parkinson's will take much longer to surface. Even worse is the fact that patients with both Parkinson's and depression can expect each condition to worsen the other.

Another way that Parkinson's opens the door for depression is by reducing the amount of serotonin in the brain. This "feel good" chemical is responsible for helping regulate your mood, but since Parkinson's actually cuts back on the supply of serotonin, you automatically become much more vulnerable to a depressive state. Serotonin is also responsible for regulating your sleep, which is another reason why Parkinson's patients have difficulty falling and remaining asleep.

But all is not lost. There are treatment options available that have proven to be very effective for many Parkinson patients. These include:

- Selective serotonin reuptake inhibitors (SSRIs). This class of antidepressants include Prozac, Zoloft and Celexa.

- Serotonin and norepinephrine reuptake inhibitors (SNRIs). Another class of antidepressants which include Cymbalta and Effexor.

- Cognitive behavioral therapy (CBT). This is a form of psychotherapy that trains the individual on how to change their mentality to think more positively and focus on those thoughts instead of fixating on negative thoughts and behaviors.

While each of these forms of treatments are effective for many, there are still those who receive little to no benefit from them. Even those who see improvement from these classes of medications may also experience some side effects. If your doctor prescribes SSRIs or SNRIs, it's vital that you closely monitor any changes that occur, both bad or good, and let them know as soon as you experience them so the necessary adjustments can be made.

Anxiety

Considering what Parkinson's patients have to deal with on a daily basis for the remainder of their lives, I guess the prevailing question is: why *wouldn't* someone with Parkinson's suffer from anxiety? After all, anytime you learn that you have a progressive, degenerative disease that has no cure, you're bound to feel anxious about your future, how the disease is going to change the quality of your life and how quickly those changes are going to take place.

Like depression, signs of anxiety tend to appear years before the physical symptoms, contributing to the notion that anxiety is a result of biological changes taking place within the brain instead of supporting the long-held theory that it is simply brought on by Parkinson's disease. The number of Parkinson's patients who experience anxiety might be lower (around 40 percent) than those of depression, but it's still a major issue with no relief in sight unless you put an identity to it and are willing to seek treatment for it. The connection between anxiety and Parkinson's is so tight that some doctors believe it could be used as a means of identifying Parkinson's in it's infancy. If this notion is true, patients could start treatment much earlier and get a better handle on the disease and potentially change their outcome substantially.

Typically, people with Parkinson's will experience anxiety due to specific fears that they have, such as the fear of falling, experiencing tremors in front of others, finding themselves in enclosed quarters (either alone or with others) or experiencing "off" times before their next dosage of medicine is due. Anxiety can even be blamed on some Parkinson medications.

Often, anxiety is more generalized, meaning it is caused by specific worries instead of being based on a broader, all-inclusive scale. When you hear the word "anxiety" being connected to an individual, undoubtedly, your first thought is that the individual is worried about something. But this is a rather simplistic approach and only a piece of the puzzle. There are actually several categories of anxiety that we, as Parkinson's patients, can experience:

1. Panic attacks. This is the most common form of anxiety, affecting approximately 1 in 3 Parkinson patients. Characteristics of this kind of anxiety can come on quickly and intensely, usually lasting a minimum of about an hour before they begin to diminish. They can be brought on by emotional distress, physical distress or both. Although they are commonly associated with "on" and "off" periods of medications, they can be brought on by any episode of intense fear or discomfort that the patient experiences.

Panic attacks bring on rapid heart rates, a shortness of breath, perspiration, dizziness, either a loss of appetite or periods of binge eating, tremors (unlike the ones associated with Parkinson's) and an intense concern for your own mortality.

2. Social avoidance. Affects roughly as much as 20 percent of

Parkinson's patients. This type of anxiety means choosing to avoid social situations either because we are afraid others will notice our condition or because we fear doing something that will embarrass us, such as tripping and/or falling, spilling a plate of food or a beverage due to shaking, etc. But these episodes are confined to the moment since the anxiety disappears once the patient is taken out of the social situation.

3. Generalized anxiety. Roughly 15 percent of Parkinson's patients have this type. Generalized means that the individual's level of anxiety is far beyond what would be considered as normal, giving an individual the hopeless feeling that they aren't in control. This type of anxiety can cause a rapid heart rate, trouble breathing, restlessness, upset stomach, inability to concentrate and a difficulty with remembering things. It can also carry over into nighttime and interrupt your sleep.

4. Obsessive compulsive disorder (OCD). This form of anxiety is characterized by unnecessary repetitive movements, thoughts or actions, such as turning a light switch on and off or locking and unlocking a door a specific number of times as a way of curtailing the anxiety.

One reason why Parkinson patients can experience more anxiety than those without the disease is due to an imbalance of certain chemicals in the brain (aside from serotonin), such as norepinephrine and, of course, dopamine. This unhealthy fluctuation causes the anxiety to morph into physical traits, such as trouble walking or a freezing gait, a more intense loss of motor skills and more dramatic "on" and "off" periods.

Other Types of Emotional Changes

Besides the predominant symptoms of depression and anxiety, there are even more emotional changes that Parkinson patients typically experience. Because Parkinson's disease is based on a disorder of both the brain and the central nervous system, it should come as no surprise that emotions will be negatively impacted and extremely heightened, even when you're dealing with the most basic of emotions.

It's realistic to think that when someone gets a diagnosis of Parkinson's disease they will experience a floodgate of emotional responses. No doubt, the person will feel a strong sense of shock and disbelief, discouragement and possibly even denial. While all of these are to be expected, that still doesn't make experiencing them healthy. All of these issues are normal, they are valid and they are very real to the individual and have to be addressed immediately or they are sure to worsen. The best way to handle them is to open up to others as much as possible instead of keeping it bottled up inside you where it can slowly eat away at your emotions. Talking to your family, as well as to your doctor, will make it much easier to deal with.

Here are some other common emotional changes that Parkinson patients are likely to go through:

1. Mood swings. Imbalances within the brain force it to become overly-sensitized to what should be standard emotions. Things that would warrant a normal reaction will become overly-exaggerated very quickly. Plus, the time it takes for the individual to fluctuate between one extreme emotion and another is dramatically shortened. Besides the hormonal shifts brought on by the disease, Parkinson sufferers could also have to contend with mood swings brought on by their medication. Compounding the problem is the fact that many caregivers, and even some doctors, unknowingly tend to overlook the behavioral issues that Parkinson patients have to contend with because they're so focused on treating the physical ones.

2. Embarrassment. Many Parkinson symptoms evoke embarrassment, not only because of how we fear we are being perceived by others, but also due to the fact that we feel so utterly helpless because we know we can't do anything about it.

It's no wonder that we feel self-conscious around others once you look at the laundry list of Parkinson symptoms that can embarrass us:

- tremors
- shuffled gait
- stooped posture
- losing our balance for no apparent reason
- low, monotone voice
- blank, stiff facial expressions
- claw deformity of hand muscles
- tremulous voice
- slow or slurred speech
- brief pauses in the middle of a sentence
- dysphagia, or difficulty swallowing
- drooling
- freezing
- trunk shaking
- dyskinesia
- dystonia

With having to focus on controlling so much all at once, feelings of embarrassment are virtually inevitable at one point or another. Besides our own challenges, these symptoms can also be brought on or made worse by our medication. At that point, it becomes a catch-22 situation because these symptoms are still guaranteed to appear whether you take the medicine or not. It can quickly turn into a balancing act where you try to determine which is the lesser of two evils, the Parkinson symptoms or the embarrassment.

3. Apathy. Having a lack of interest in participating in things- even things that are part of your daily routine- is very common for Parkinson patients, affecting upwards of 60 percent of them- even those who are in the early stages of the disease. In fact, apathy often manifests earlier than when a person receives their diagnosis.

Having a feeling of apathy makes it difficult- and sometimes, even impossible- to become interested in doing your normal activities. In some cases, the apathetic individual can even have great difficulty being motivated just to get out of bed. Besides having a lack of interest, those with apathy also find it increasingly difficult to initiate, continue or complete tasks that, under normal conditions, would not warrant that kind of an effort.

Apathy can also surface as feeling a lack of concern for yourself and those around you- even your loved ones. How much you care about others isn't being called into question here because everyone understands that this nothing more than a ramification of the disease and not who you really are so it's important for allowances to be made.

There are several ways that you can combat apathy and gain some, if not all, of that part of your life back:

- List out the activities that you want, or need, to get accomplished.
- Set a mandatory completion date for them.
- Log these activities somewhere highly-visible that will guarantee you'll keep up with them.
- As you complete a task, mark it off and reward yourself in some way.
- If you still find it difficult to stick to a schedule, ask someone to hold you accountable.

4. Feeling "blue". Despite what some people may believe, feeling blue is *not* the same thing as being depressed. Feeling blue refers to someone who is sad or lacks interest in normal activities while depression is an extreme case of "the blues". Another major difference is that someone who is blue can overcome their sadness in time just by learning to cope with what they're feeling while depression can last for long periods of time and most likely will require some type of outside assistance in order in order for you to effectively deal with it.

How Parkinson's Affects Your Memory and Other Brain Functions

Since Parkinson's disease originates within the brain it's perfectly understandable for patients to be concerned about how the disease will affect their mental faculties. While there is a legitimate reason for concern- to an extent- it should not be an overwhelming concern that you should begin to fixate on since you could easily cause yourself more anxiety than the situation calls for.

Once an individual has been diagnosed with Parkinson's, the average person can typically expect to remain mentally unscathed during the early stages of the disease, as long as they take care of themselves and exercise on a regular basis. In fact, these leveling-off periods often do extend for many years without witnessing any significant changes. It's only as the disease progresses that these changes to brain function begin to occur. Although some of these changes are normal for someone with Parkinson's, there are still lifestyle changes that you can make to help prolong the amount of time before they begin to be a concern.

Even though Parkinson's disease and Alzheimer's disease are both neurological degenerative disorders, the cognitive problems associated with Parkinson's are different than those of Alzheimer's and typically only affect less than 15 percent of all Parkinson patients. Sadly, over time, the vast majority of patients will eventually end up with some type of decline in cognitive behavior, but that doesn't mean that it can always be blamed on Parkinson's. Since a large number of non-Parkinson individuals typically develop some form of cognitive decline anyway, it's often difficult to assess whether the decline can be blamed on Parkinson's or if it is just the natural course of events that has nothing to do with the disease and would have taken place, regardless.

The downside to this fact is that having Parkinson's disease does put patients at an increased risk of experiencing cognitive problems. These patients can expect to see difficulty with planning and organizing, multitasking, keeping up with conversations involving more than a few people at once and paying attention. The good news is that Parkinson patients rarely have to worry about developing memory loss or the decline of their cognitive faculties in the same way that Alzheimer's patients are prone to developing. Even if they do, they will be minor in comparison to those of Alzheimer's and won't begin to appear until many years later during the latter stages of Parkinson's.

Hallucinations

Otherwise known as "psychosis", hallucinations affects roughly 1 in every 5 Parkinson's' patients at some point. Much more minor forms of hallucinations, such as your eyes tricking you into believing you're seeing something for an instant that isn't really there happens much more frequently, roughly in 2 out of every 3 patients. These "split-second" sightings often go unnoticed or are easily dismissed since many older non-Parkinson individuals can also experience them, as well.

But hallucinations don't always have to be visual in nature. About 10-20 percent of Parkinson patients experience hallucinations, which are audible in nature. These are also easily dismissed since they are only temporary and, as a result, fail to illicit any permanent persuasion to what you hear around you.

Unfortunately, those with hallucinations can expect them to increase in frequency, as well as severity, as Parkinson's disease progresses. This increase can also be brought on by other factors, including sleep deprivation and, ironically, your Parkinson medications. As the patient gets older and the disease progresses into later stages, the brain becomes more delicate and episodes of psychosis can be brought on by something as simple as stress. What we might perceive to be standard life issues can become major concerns for those with advanced Parkinson's.

The most common form of psychosis in advanced cases of Parkinson's targets spouses or other types of caregiver. The patient will begin to feel paranoia that their caregiver (be it a spouse or someone who is not related to them) is trying to inflict harm on them in some manner, ranging from something as simple as the individual stealing from them to much more severe thoughts, such as the belief that the caregiver is plotting to kill them. As time passes, the psychosis becomes much more severe and real to the patient, requiring medication to ease the distress to prevent them for hurting themselves or someone else out of desperation. At a certain point, the patient becomes so consumed with the psychosis that they are no longer able to distinguish between fantasy and reality.

It should be mentioned that psychosis can be the result of a medical condition, such as an infection or it can also be brought on by a reaction to specific medications- even those prescribed to treat Parkinson's. Sometimes, a doctor will be forced to temporarily halt the administering of these medications in an effort to ease psychosis symptoms, depending on how debilitating the psychosis becomes and how much of a danger they are being placed in. This is one area in particular where a caregiver's observations can be very helpful.

Chapter 7

How Diet Affects Parkinson's (You'll Be Surprised)

By now, you've been given a virtual laundry list of ways that Parkinson's disease makes your life a living nightmare. If you have already been diagnosed, then you already know about them. If you haven't received a diagnosis, think of this as a tool to prepare you for the future.

Almost all of these issues are things that are completely out of our hands, leaving us with no other choice but to accept them as fact, learn how to deal with them as best we can and do whatever we can to limit the amount of influence they hold over the quality of our lives. But what if I told you that there were actually some things that you *did* have complete control over that also determine, within reason, how you will feel and the severity of your symptoms? Well, there is. It's the food that you eat.

As humans, it's in our nature to want to exercise our right to free will. Believe me, of all people, I get that. We rebel even when we know it isn't necessarily the right decision to make simply because we can and we don't hesitate to implement that right anytime it can benefit us in some way.

It isn't a matter of knowledge or even common sense. It always comes down to a choice. We know that an apple is better for us than a cheeseburger. We know that a serving of blueberries is a better option than a bowl of ice cream. We know this and, yet, we choose to ignore the rationality. We make bad choices not because we don't care about our health but because we *want* the cheeseburger and we *want* the ice cream, so we eat it, knowing that there are going to be consequences to our health as a result. Since those consequences don't outweigh the reward we put those realities out of our minds, for the time being, and indulge in what brings us pleasure.

When we're young, we can get away with making illogical decisions about the things we eat because we feel as if we're invincible and our bodies haven't begun to feel the effects of long-term abuse from food. But as we age, our bodies start to revolt and the years of self-sabotage begin to take their toll on our health until we can no longer ignore the blatant truth. Most people, myself included, still ignore the signs as long as we can get away with it. For some, once again myself included, it takes contracting a serious illness like Parkinson's disease before they realize they are never going to be able to beat reality. As much as we would like to feel triumphant over food, it's a battle we're going to lose each and every time. Eventually, the food you eat (or don't eat) will catch up to you. It's a certainty that you can count on just like the sun rising in the morning.

While maintaining a proper, balanced diet is important for everyone, it's of particular importance for those with Parkinson's. The food that you consume can either offer you a tremendous boost to your health and a reduction in your symptoms or it can turn a bad situation into a horrible one. It's your choice.

There might not be a specific diet that can magically make your disease go away- albeit temporary- but there are plenty of thing that you can do to ensure that you receive the maximize benefits from the proper foods. And those benefits not only feed your body the vital vitamins, minerals and nutrients that it was designed by nature to run on in the first place, but they also help you get a better grip on your disease. Who cares if the improvements are only temporary? All you have to do to prolong those improvements is to continue eating the right foods meal after meal.

Why You Need To Eat Regular Meals

One of the biggest problems facing everyone- not just Parkinson patients- is the fact that we skip meals. It might seem rational to assume that avoiding a meal would help us to lose weight or to at least maintain our current weight- assuming weight loss wasn't a goal of yours. But if this is your mindset, then you should know that this kind of assumption would be wrong.

We are designed to receive fuel on a regular basis- not sporadically. Our bodies work like a propeller on an airplane: while fuel is being supplied to run the propeller, everything is fine. But once you shut off the supply of fuel that keeps it going, you're in big trouble. We would hesitate to cut off the fuel supply to an airplane in flight, but we never think twice about the effects we will reap as a result of cutting off our body's fuel supply. The same should hold true for us. We weren't meant to go long stretches of time without food. When we do, we're going against our design and, as a result, we have to face the consequences.

Take breakfast, for example. If you go to bed at, say, eleven o'clock and typically eat breakfast at seven o'clock, you're coming off of an 8-hour forced fast. There's nothing you can do about providing your body fuel while you're sleeping, but that's okay because if you planned your dinner properly you should be providing sufficient fuel for it to run it's primary systems while you sleep. However, there is something you can do about it once you get up and it's called breakfast. You may feel sluggish and run down when you rise (which is completely understandable), but if you have breakfast- specifically the right kind of breakfast, your body will not only bounce back, but it'll do it quicker and easier *and* give you enough fuel to run off of until lunch.

On the other hand, if you choose to skip breakfast and wait until you eat lunch at noon, you're extending your fast for another 5 hours, for a total of 13 hours. That's 13 hours that you have intentionally deprived your body of much-needed fuel. That's also well beyond the time frame that it will allow you to provide it more fuel. So what does it do in retaliation to your deprivation? It shuts down your metabolism.

Once your body reaches a certain point without receiving food, it begins to panic because it's unsure when, or if, you're going to eat again. In response, your body turns your metabolism way down, retreating into what is appropriately called "starvation mode". You might be saving yourself a few calories by missing a meal, but in the process you're also virtually shutting down the burning of fat. Not only that, but now that your metabolism has been forced into survival mode, it will be thrown off-balance for the rest of the day, whereas eating breakfast does just the opposite and stokes your metabolism till bedtime. In short, you've started the day off wrong and it's something that your body doesn't easily forget.

How Protein Affects Parkinson's

No one can argue the fact that we all need protein- especially bodybuilders who swear by consuming large quantities of it in order to achieve their massive gains or in smaller amounts for those who are just looking to trim and tone. In fact, it's the second-most commonly found item in our bodies after water. But protein is so much more than just a physique enhancer or a source of fuel for the body. It's one of the most important amino acids that you can take in. Yet, as far as protein goes, Parkinson patients are faced with the dilemma that we have to both respect it and fear it at the same time.

Protein is responsible for building muscle tissue, reducing fat (since muscle burns more calories than fat), improving blood pressure, boosting your immune system, improving your sleep and helping keep you fuller, longer so you have an extended level of energy. Not only is it also important in the building of hair, nails, bone, skin and cells, but when you take into account how it aids in the workings of enzymes, that alone encompasses virtually every function of the body. It also helps strengthen tendons, which is a big plus for Parkinson patients who need as much help stabilizing their walking as possible.

The chemical changes within the brain and the bodily functions that take place within our bodies are all due to hormones and enzymes made possible by the power of protein. Our brains benefit greatly from protein because it supplies the brain with several components, such as:

Creatine- helps to supply energy to cells- especially muscle (although it can be found in trace amounts in some fruits, vegetables and carbs, it is primarily only found in meat and some seafood).

Carnosine- contains powerful antioxidant properties, such as the ability to offer protection against oxidative stress (only found in the meat and, if you can stomach it, the brains of animals).

Protein is also loaded with some other important compounds:

- Omega-3 fatty acids- provides tons of protection for your cardiovascular system
- Vitamin B12
- Vitamin D

As you can see, protein plays many vital roles in our lives. Now, the bad news about protein, or the next thing I wish I had known when I was first diagnosed:

Insight #4: Protein often affects your medication.

We all know that when you eat protein versus carbs, for example, you're going to feel more energized and alert- unless you overindulge, that is. But Parkinson's patients have a unique situation when it comes to eating protein because having too much of it or having it at the wrong times can interfere with their medications. Although the problem typically becomes more pronounced in patients who have advanced into the middle or end stages of the disease, early-stage patients can easily experience it, too.

How can protein pose such a threat while still offering us so many benefits? Because one group of amino acids found in protein, called large neutral amino acids (LNAA), actually compete with Levodopa and intercepts it from getting into our brains where it can be made into Dopamine. Protein also interferes with how Levodopa is absorbed into the bloodstream. This was disheartening news for me because I grew up in the South where I was raised as a "meat and potatoes" kind of guy so I've always centered my meals around ample amounts of protein followed by scant amounts of everything else. Unbeknownst to me, that little seemingly-harmless habit that had been instilled in me since childhood was now coming back to haunt me by interfering with my medication's ability of being able to do its intended job. In the beginning, I didn't know that and I paid the price through a worsening of symptoms without even realizing that I was doing it to myself.

It is recommended that you limit your intake of protein while you're taking Carbidopa/Levodopa as it will severely negate the effects of the medication. If you are a diehard meat person and are determined to eat protein with your meals, do yourself a favor and at least try to cut down your portion sizes, as much as possible, while still satisfying your cravings. The less protein you consume, the less you're jeopardizing the effects of your medication.

What causes this interaction between dopamine and protein? It all has to do with the small intestines. Dopamine uses special carriers to transport itself across the small intestines into the bloodstream where it can be best utilized. Unfortunately, protein uses the same highway so the two compete against one another for the same ride, like two people fighting to ride the same bicycle, all the while minimizing the level of dopamine that you're receiving, as well as lowering its effectiveness.

But as bad as the protein situation sounds there's a group that poses an even bigger threat to dopamine absorption. They're called branched-chain amino acids, or BCAAs. Three BCAAs in particular, Leucine, Valine and Isoleucine, all directly interfere with the absorption of Levodopa- even more than your typical protein amino acids. Where are BCAAs prevalent? The list of BCAA foods to be on the lookout for include red meat, chicken and poultry, fish, dairy and eggs. For the super-health conscience individuals who like to supplement their protein through shakes and smoothies, BCAAs can also be found in whey supplements and protein powders.

But don't just focus on your meat intake. In order to fully protect yourself, you need to be aware that protein isn't just limited to meats and dairy: some fruits and vegetables contain significant levels of protein, too. Vegetables to be on the lookout for include:

- peas and lentils
- mushrooms
- sweet corn
- artichokes

- green, leafy vegetables
- broccoli
- asparagus

As for fruits, the list includes:

- bananas
- avocado
- guavas
- apricots
- grapefruit
- cantaloupe
- peaches
- oranges
- pomegranate

Instead of crossing protein out of your meals completely, a better option for consuming protein is to take it at least 30 minutes before or at least one and preferably up to two hours after a meal. But the best option, by far, is to limit your intake of protein throughout the day as much as possible so you don't have to worry about keeping up with the timing. Recommendations are to limit your total daily intake of protein to around 7 ounces and to postpone eating protein until the last meal of the day.

Other things that interfere with Carbidopa/Levodopa absorption are iron supplements, specific kinds of Parkinson medications and some psychiatric and antidepressant medicines so make sure to take all of those into account, too.

Lastly, for those who have only been prescribed Levodopa, you should be cautious taking vitamin B6 or any supplements containing vitamin B6 as it has been shown to reduce the effects of the medication.

The Ketogenic Diet

Some Parkinson patients have switched up their eating style in favor of a more regimented program, such as the Ketogenic diet. This program (I hesitate to actually call it a diet since it is primarily a way of life for those who decide to adopt it long-term) is an eating plan which focuses on three areas:

- high amounts of fat
- moderate amounts of protein
- low amounts of carbs

The Ketogenic diet was originally created a century ago to treat the seizures in epileptic children- which it did quite well, I might add. It closely mirrors today's infamous Atkins diet, which pushes high amounts of protein, and thus, higher amounts of fat. It is because of this allowance of more meats and fats that has made the Atkins diet so popular.

The purpose of the Ketogenic eating plan is to force the body to burn fat instead of burning carbs like it naturally wants to. In a typical eating situation, the body grabs the carbs that we take in, converts them over into glucose and then carries them throughout the body to the various areas where they are needed. But in the Ketogenic plan, the body is forced to switch things up, providing you with a 4:1 ratio of fat to a combination of both protein and carbs. Since there are only small amounts of carbs available, the body is encouraged to hold them in reserves and instead to turn to fat for its energy needs.

The liver taps into the ample supply of fat that you're giving it and converts it over to fatty acids and ketone bodies. Ketone bodies are water-soluble molecules that the liver makes from fatty acids that are used for energy in the place of glucose. These are made when the body is not receiving what it feels is an ample supply of carbs. When the amount of ketone bodies in the blood increase, this creates a condition known as ketosis.

If you are discouraged by the limitations that this plan imposes or feel that you might have difficulty living up to its parameters there are other variations of the Ketogenic plan that allow for some changes to be made. One version that many people choose to follow is called the medium-chain triglycerides or MCT Ketogenic diet. This version focuses on the use of coconut oil, which ends up providing approximately half of your calories. By limiting your total fat intake, it opens up more choices for carbs and proteins, adding additional food choices to the mix.

But while the Ketogenic program might seem like a dream come true for meat-lovers, there is a catch. In order to prevent your ketone bodies from becoming too elevated, it is necessary for the patient to test their urine to ensure that ketone levels are kept within acceptable limits. This is done using a ketone screening kit, requiring you to urinate on a test strip. The color indicated is then matched to the corresponding color on the provided color chart to determine ketone levels. If levels become too high, you will develop a condition known as ketonuria, which can become very serious so it's important to routinely monitor this.

Plant-based diets

We've all heard the phrase "you are what you eat". Remember that after you've read what I'm about to share with you.

I'm giving you fair warning that this next section might be a little disturbing for some to read because I'm about to share the truth concerning what happens to us when we consume animal protein. I want to go on record as saying that I'm not trying to use scare tactics to force you to give up animal protein, but at the same time I think everyone needs to know what they're eating when we ingest your typical animal protein. If you feel like you might be a little squeamish about the subject and want to skip this section altogether, I completely understand.

Now, let's talk about animal protein.

Only a few, short decades ago, the Atkins diet was the latest rage. People loved the idea of this eating plan because it meant that you could have virtuously limitless amounts of animal protein and lots and lots of fat. Suppressed meat-eaters everywhere who had been forced to succumb to the tight restrictions of a typical diet for so many years were finally set free and able to indulge in massive amounts of their favorite meats to their heart's content. After all, it was an ideal situation for all of us meat lovers, right?

Well, not exactly.

The harmful effects that animal protein inflicts on the body are nothing new. There is more and more research constantly being conducted about the harm of consuming animal proteins and, subsequently, the effectiveness of a plant-based diet on Parkinson's symptoms, with the results being nothing short of extraordinary (I'll get to that in a second). First, I need to discuss animal proteins.

You see, when you eat animal protein, there's so much more that you need to be concerned about than just the calories and the fat content, which, of course, are also important points that shouldn't be overlooked, either.

As far as beef, pork and poultry goes, you have to worry about the things that farmers add to their feed in order to maximize results, expedite growth and make the farmer more money. These additives include but are not limited to such things as growth hormones, antibiotics and steroids, for example. You have to worry about the very food that the animal was fed, including genetically-engineered crops (such as corn) and, believe it or not, a disgusting combination of uneaten chicken food, chicken feathers and chicken poop (that's right, chicken *poop*) affectionately named "poultry litter" or "chicken litter" (I kid you not: if you don't believe me, by all means, Google it. The first time I read it I couldn't believe it myself).

I hope you're not thoroughly disgusted because there's more. As a way to cut costs, cattle are often fed bone meal and waste products from other cattle, in other words, the parts of a cow that can't be cut up and sold as food products. This would be disturbing enough if it weren't for the fact that this is typically how Bovine Spongiform Encepholopathy (BSE), otherwise known as "mad cow disease", is transmitted, an illness that results in progressive dementia and death, typically in about a year after exposure.

Another issue is the fact that legislation was recently approved that states meat distributors no longer have to identify the country of origin on their products. What does this mean? It means that grocery stores can buy meat and not have to be concerned where the animal was raised. This is of importance for consumers because most foreign countries don't have nearly the health standards as we do. That, in itself is an alarming statement considering that the Food and Drug Administration (FDA) has very lax standards of their own concerning meat and what is allowed to be present in it, how it can be raised and what it can be fed. So just imagine how much looser the standards of an undeveloped country are. It's probably not something you want to think about too much.

But that still isn't everything. If you think you're safe by eliminating land-based animals and choosing to get your protein from the oceans, I'm here to tell you that this isn't a safe approach, either. There's the damage your body is subjected to as a result of heavy metals found in fish and other seafood (namely mercury) plus the fact that, in either case, if you're downing a considerable amount of animal proteins it's more than likely that you're *not* downing a significant amount of fresh fruits and vegetables. That means you're depriving yourself of very important phytonutrients and antioxidants designed by nature to provide an umbrella of protection for your immune system and your body's overall health.

As I mentioned at the beginning of this section, there has been scientific documentation that a plant-based diet is quite beneficial for Parkinson patients, even though people tend to shy away from this option because they feel that they just can't go through life without meat. I know because I have a hard time cutting back on my consumption of animal protein- even knowing what I now know. That still doesn't make it right and I'm hoping one day soon I'll wake up, realize what I'm really putting into my body and make the decision to go completely plant-based. But for now, it's something I'm still working on. If you're in this group, that's okay. Plant-Based diets aren't for everyone. I just felt compelled to share with you what goes into animal protein before it hits your grocery store shelves.

While I have read different studies on the subject, there was one study, in particular, concerning plant-based diets, which caught my attention. It involved a 53-year old dietician who developed

Parkinson's disease back in 2000 and, in the beginning, decided to follow something known as a "protein redistribution plan". The goal was to limit animal protein to just the evening meal in the hopes that the negative effects of the protein would wear off enough by the time the individual went to bed. This diet consisted of mostly fruits, vegetables, extra-virgin olive oil, nonfat milk products, nuts, seeds, 100 whole grains and small amounts of dark chocolate, with no more than 25 g of animal fat each day. She was cutting back on meat, but, as you can see, she was still getting an ample supply of dairy.

For the next nine years, her symptoms continued as before. Then, during a follow-up visit to her neurologist in 2009, her doctor suggested that she switch her diet over to one that was completely plant-based, with particular focus on increasing levels of two phytonutrients, fisetin, a flavonol found in most fruits and vegetables (including the skin of cucumbers) and n-hexacosanol, a long-chain fatty alcohol found in some vegetable and fruit peels (such as cabbage, for example). To this date, there haven't been many studies which focused on these two particular phytonutrients, but her doctor just happened to specifically name them, feeling that it would be a good starting point.

Six months later on another follow-up visit, her doctor noticed a significant improvement in her symptoms. According to the report,

"...the patient's attending neurologist observed an almost complete absence of the previous cog-wheel rigidity, miccrographia, bradykinesis, dystonia, constricted arm swing with gait, hypomimia (lack of facial expression) and retropulsion (a tendency to lose your balance leaning backwards)."

Unfortunately, there was little improvement in her tremors, but, at this point, I'll take what I can get. I know this is only one person, but you can't argue with those kind of results.

I didn't tell you all of this to make you swear off animal protein. And no, I don't have an axe to grind with the beef industry, the chicken industry, the pork council or the dairy industry, but facts are facts- no matter how disturbing they might be. It just stands to reason that when you ingest food that contains

- growth hormones
- antibiotics
- steroids
- genetically-modified feed
- chicken litter
- bone meal
- waste products
- mercury
  and
- iron/other heavy metals

you can't really be expected to be surprised when your health suffers. And since studies have shown how animal proteins actually block how L-dopa is transported into the brain, you not only have to be concerned about what's in your animal protein, but you also have to contend with the fact that it is actually undermining what you're working towards, which is an increase in L-dopa. In other words, we're taking medication to increase L-dopa levels and then trying to undo everything by eating animal protein.

In another study conducted a few years ago in Italy, it was proven that a plant-based diet boosts L-dopa levels. Besides the obvious reason just mentioned, here's what the resulting report stated:

"Thanks to its characteristics, a plant-based diet, particularly in its vegan variant, is expected to raise levodopa bioavailability and bring some advantages in the management of the disease through two mechanisms: a reduced protein intake and an increased fiber intake (in comparison to an omnivorous diet (OD)). In fact, protein-rich plant food (namely legumes and nuts), also provide fiber, in contrast to animal food."

The results of this study were clear. When Parkinson patients were placed on a vegan diet, with the main stipulation being that they put off their consumption of beans until the end of the day, there was a significant improvement in symptoms because L-dopa was allowed to do its job unscathed.

Blood Sugar

Besides trashing your metabolism, do you know what else happens to you when you skip a meal? Your blood sugar drops. You might think this isn't a problem unless you happen to be diabetic, but that's simply not the case. Everyone is affected by a drop in blood sugar, but it's just that for some the effects are more visible than for others. Low blood sugar can make you feel lethargic, lightheaded, dizzy, sleepy, have difficulty concentrating and give you tremors, all of which mirror the symptoms of Parkinson's disease.

You also have to be on the lookout for trouble from the other end of the spectrum, or high blood sugar. When blood sugar levels become elevated due to a poor diet, consuming too much sugar and simple carbs, lack of exercise or any combination of the three, it means that the body can't produce enough insulin to keep up with demand. Since something has to give in this scenario, the excess sugar is left roaming around in your body, creating havoc in a lot of places because it's nestling in areas that it has no business being. One of the first places it affects just happens to be your feet.

Now this is important because when you subject your extremities to elevated blood sugar for extended periods of time, the sugar begins to damage the nerves, a condition known as neuropathy. This condition is characterized by a tingling, aching or a numbing of parts of the foot of possibly even the entire foot. Eventually, these nerves are subjected to so much trauma that it kills them. Up until the time that the nerves become completed destroyed, the Parkinson patient has to deal with an increase of an unsteady posture because they can no longer rely on their feet to steady them. Anyone with Parkinson's will tell you that the last thing they want to lose is their balance.

The reality of having elevated blood sugar is that many individuals aren't aware of it, putting themselves in even greater danger because they're unknowingly causing damage to themselves without treating the issue. Over time, this damage will become irreparable and, at a certain point, it requires amputation of either part of the foot or the entire foot, depending on the extent of the damage.

But the problem with elevated sugar doesn't stop there. Did you know that type 2 diabetics are at a 40 percent higher risk of also developing Parkinson's? You might think this is irrelevant if you already have Parkinson's, but it wouldn't be too late for your family and friends to know. Maybe sharing this with them could significantly reduce their chances of developing Parkinson's. With both of my parents being diabetic, which increases my risk of also becoming diabetic, I've often wondered if that had an influence on my getting Parkinson's.

But let's say you already have Parkinson's, which is a fair assumption since you're reading this book, so you aren't really concerned about diabetes at this point. That doesn't mean that you're completely out of the woods. Did you know that having diabetes *doubles* your risk of also developing Alzheimer's disease, the very same disease whose risk is already increased by having Parkinson's? *That's* something to think about.

How Sugar Complicates Parkinson's

It's hard to get away from sugar because it's everywhere and in virtually everything. But the reason it's all around us is because we can never seem to get enough of it. The fact is, we truly do love the white stuff, despite the fact that the white stuff is literally killing us.

Consider the fact that less than a hundred years ago, the average person ingested just 4 pounds of sugar in a year. Not bad, right? Today, that average has skyrocketed to 170 pounds per year, or roughly half-a pound per day. And that's just an *average*. Statistics show that some people eat an unbelievable 300 pounds of sugar in one year. That's almost a pound of sugar *every day*! It's no wonder diabetes is sweeping across the globe at an unprecedented rate.

It probably doesn't surprise you that sugar has been labeled as being addictive, but do you know just how addictive it really is? These facts might surprise you.

There have been numerous studies where rats were fed cocaine and sugar at different times. Later, when the rats were exposed to both cocaine and sugar at the same time, the rats consistently chose the sugar. Sugar over cocaine. Who knew?

When we eat sugar, the part of our brain known as the Nucleus Accumbens releases a chemical as a reward for being fed a treat. What's the name of that chemical? Dopamine. But over time, the constant barrage of sugar entering our body begins to wear at and, in essence, eat away at the brain, desensitizing the receptors that are responsible for releasing the dopamine. So the next time you eat sugar, there are fewer receptors to intercept this reaction, which means you'll have to take in even more sugar to achieve the same level of satisfaction as you have in the past. Enter cravings.

Now, we add Parkinson's into the mix, a disease that is known for actually destroying dopamine levels. That means that not only are there now fewer dopamine receptors to illicit a response to the sugar, but the ones that are there are becoming more and more immune to the effects of the sugar. It's a lose-lose situation.

Sugar has been *proven* to have the same effects on the reward system of our brains as cocaine, nicotine and alcohol, which is why all three are considered to be addictive. We always hear about how dangerous these substances are, how addictive they can become and how easily and quickly that can occur, but how ironic is it that we never hear about the similar dangers of sugar, which falls into the same addictive category. That's not to mention the fact that increased sugar consumption means a dramatic increase in your risk of developing type 2 diabetes, heart disease or having a stroke.

Now, consider the connection between sugar and Alzheimer's disease, a disease that now affects one in every 9 people over the age of 65 and has become the third-highest cause of death following heart disease and cancer. We know that Parkinson patients are more susceptible to developing Alzheimer's, but you might not know that there are several facts that point out how much sugar can affect that outcome.

Up until just recently, it's been well-known for years that type 2 diabetics tend to lose more brain volume than non-diabetics. But now that volume loss has been increased even more- including the precious "gray matter" that ups your risk of developing dementia.

Another issue is the fact that scientists have only discovered within the last decade that the pancreas is not the only organ in the body that produces insulin: so does the brain. It is this brain insulin that helps regulate neurotransmitters while also ensuring that neurons receive glucose. But when your sugar levels are off, so is this delicate brain/insulin balance, which leads to cognitive issues.

The bottom line is that sugar affects your brain even if you aren't diabetic or even pre-diabetic. Short-term, it disrupts your memory and cognitive skills. Long-term, it jeopardizes the health of the hippocampus part of your brain (the part that deals with every aspect of memories, from creating them to storing them), which also just so happens to be a classic pre-requisite to Alzheimer's.

This was especially troubling news for me since I have had a life-long struggle with sugar. Growing up, our house was always overflowing with cookies, cakes and pies to satisfy our insatiable cravings for sugar. But my Achilles' heel has always been my weakness for sweet tea, the one and only drink that ever graced our tables each time we sat down to graze. Many years later, I found out that I not only had to be concerned with the sugar intake, but now that I had Parkinson's, I also had another concern, which brought me to the next thing I wish I had known when I was first diagnosed:

Insight #5: Caffeine can (in some cases) make your symptoms worse.

While there are some scientists who theorize that caffeine may actually help to reduce the risk of developing Parkinson's disease, that doesn't really offer help to those of us who have already been diagnosed. Or does it?

Studies conducted all over the world in Germany, Spain and Sweden, dating all the way back to 1968, appear to show numerous instances where coffee drinkers were able to delay the onset of Parkinson's disease simply by their regular consumption of caffeine. Scientists have since learned that this is possible, again only in some cases, because caffeine works in the same way as D2 dopaminergic receptors by offering protection to neurons while reducing the degeneration of dopaminergic cells.

There have also been different studies conducted to determine just how caffeine is able to help those of us who already have Parkinson's. Given the association between the disease and tremors, and knowing full-well the usual affects that caffeine has on our bodies by increasing blood flow and adrenaline, it might seem counterproductive to give an artificial stimulant to someone who is already battling tremors. But you might be surprised to know that doing so is not only considered by some as being safe, but it is also recommended.

In some cases, these studies have shown that caffeine not only improves motor skills in certain individuals with Parkinson's, but it also appears to improve their general mobility, as well as reducing the severity of the individual's tremors. The problem is researchers also noted that the reduction of these symptoms that caffeine offers tends to lessen over time. Still, it's a fascinating concept. So how is caffeine able to accomplish this in these instances when it is theoretically supposed to make matters worse?

It's all because of a component found in the central nervous system called adenosine A2A receptors. Adenosine, a neurotransmitter, naturally dilates the blood vessels to slow down neurological activity and induce a relaxed, sleepy feeling. Along with D2 dopaminergic receptors located in the cerebral region of the brain known as the striatum, these A2A receptors are partially and temporarily blocked by the effects of caffeine, allowing for a greater range of motor activities while simultaneously reducing the amount of motor deficits. Once caffeine is present in these adenosine receptors, it not only interferes with this sedation, but it also entices the pituitary gland to persuade the adrenal gland into increasing adrenaline production.

Caffeine also causes the brain to ramp up its production of dopamine. But while all of this might sound rather appealing, especially if you suffer from low energy, you still have to accept the fact that caffeine, like any other type of artificial stimulant, has to be respected. This is not one of those cases where "more is better". You can have too much of a good thing and while caffeine may offer you some temporary relief, it can still cause a Parkinson patient to experience the jitters just as easily as it can someone who doesn't have Parkinson's. In other words, moderation is the key.

Cholesterol

For decades, cholesterol has been portrayed as the villain responsible for so much heart disease and early death. But then, on the other hand, over 60 percent of your brain is made up of fat. Coincidence? Not hardly. Is it because we consume a diet too high in fat, forcing a majority of that fat to collect in our brains and build to dangerous levels? Not exactly.

We've not only been told our entire lives that it isn't enough just to keep our cholesterol levels down as much as possible in order to promote a healthier, happier lifestyle, but it's been pounded into our heads that we should avoid it like the plaque. In fact, the prevailing word has always been that the lower we could get our cholesterol down to, the better off we are and the healthier we would be. Sound familiar?

Now, doctors have been forced to change their minds.

It seems they've now realized that all the negative hype that they generated surrounding the evils of cholesterol was going quite a bit overboard. They have been forced to admit that not only was cholesterol not as evil as they had made it out to be, but that it actually served a valuable purpose. What caused such a radical change of heart (no pun intended)? Get ready because you're going to love this. Researchers discovered that low cholesterol levels can significantly contribute to the likelihood of developing Parkinson's. That's the point behind the next thing I wish I'd known when I was first diagnosed:

Insight #6: It's important to keep your cholesterol levels *up*.

This is going to be a hard concept for some to grasp because it goes against everything we've ever been told by the medical community. Instead of continuing to take the old news about cholesterol as being law, scientists decided that they had to get to the bottom of what was causing the number of cases of Parkinson's disease to continue to skyrocket year after year without any clear indicators flagging their attention. Something had to be done to help determine why Parkinson's was becoming so prevalent and it had to be done quickly.

They took it upon themselves to start conducting numerous studies to try to figure out why so many people were developing Parkinson's disease in the first place when there appeared to be no obvious causes for the increase. This meant that the increase had to be due to a hidden factor that everyone was overlooking. They were right. The results they found were shocking, to say the least. Why? Because for the first time ever, they discovered irrefutable proof that there was an obvious connection between low cholesterol and the occurrence of Parkinson's disease. You read that right: *low* cholesterol.

For decades, no one dared to challenge the status quo. We took the details concerning cholesterol as the truth, the whole truth and nothing but the truth without ever looking back or questioning it. But a collaborative study by researchers from Harvard and Pennsylvania State University is just the latest of news outpourings that has shown us how low levels of cholesterol not only plays a role but a significant role in the progression of Parkinson's.

It turns out that cholesterol isn't as evil as it has always been made out to be. Besides helping to protect the brain from the harmful effects of free radicals by offering it a shield of antioxidant protection, cholesterol also serves as the precursor to many of the brain's most important hormones including estrogen, testosterone and vitamin D.

One such study performed at the University of North Carolina at

Chapel Hill showed that men who have a cholesterol level between 91 and 135 were *six times* as likely to develop Parkinson's disease. They also found that men who were super-vigilant about their cholesterol and managed to get it down even further, say below 91, weren't doing themselves any favors, either, because even they were *four* times as likely to get Parkinson's. But low cholesterol doesn't seem to only be a risk factor for Parkinson's because turns out it affects other conditions, too. Having an imbalance of cholesterol also increases your risk of developing other types of neurological disorders including Huntington's disease.

So what is the connection here? Why is something that is seemingly supposed to be so bad for us actually a good thing? It all comes back to why we should have cholesterol in the first place. The fact is that our brains need two types of fats, saturated fat and cholesterol, in order to be classified as being "healthy". This isn't just a suggestion but more like a requirement if we want to maintain a healthy brain.

The reason why one-quarter of the cholesterol in your body can be found in the brain is because it is necessary in order for it to perform a number of functions:

- it helps remove toxins from your brain
- it's critical for membrane function
- it serves as the building block for the creation of important hormones such as estrogen, progesterone, cortisol and testosterone
- it's responsible for manufacturing vitamin D

Science shows us that up to 90 percent of the cholesterol in our central nervous system is located in the myelin, which is the insulating layer that surrounds our nerves, particularly those located in the spinal cord and the brain. The purpose of the myelin is to allow the transmission of electrical signals and it is necessary for your nervous system to perform properly.

I know about this first-hand. I found out that my cholesterol was too low and it was causing my symptoms to be much worse than they needed to be. Plus, I found out that there were other things in my diet that were contributing to the progression of my Parkinson's. I'll cover those more in detail in Chapter 8.

But as hard of a time as I was having with trying to get my Parkinson's under control, I would soon find out that I had much more pressing things to worry about.

On December 19, 2013, a little over two months since I was diagnosed, I was still trying to get a firm grasp on Parkinson's and what I was up against. I remember it was a normal, cool afternoon and I was out with my family. We were standing in a parking lot talking with my mother-in-law when I began to feel as if my right foot was falling asleep. I took a few steps away from the group and tried to walk it off, but the more steps I took, the more my foot wasn't cooperating. Suddenly, I realized my entire right leg was dragging. Since I couldn't put any weight on my leg I tried to reach up with my right arm to catch myself against my car for balance and that's when I realized that my right arm wouldn't move.

I was having a stroke.

I panicked. I tried to catch myself with my left arm as the front of my body fell flat against the side of my SUV. I tried to call my wife's name, but all I could manage to speak was faint, garbled muttering. My wife looked over and, at first, thought I was clowning around, but then when she saw that I was struggling just to remain standing she realized that something was definitely wrong. My wife and mother-in-law had to help me into the back seat of our car while they dialed 9-1-1.

Fortunately, we were only about a mile from the nearest fire station. As I was waiting for the ambulance to arrive, my 14-year-old daughter was sitting next to me, holding my hand and crying. She was asking me to try to squeeze her hand to show her some kind of response, but I couldn't make it happen no matter who hard I tried. She was trying to be brave and hold herself together as much as possible, but each time I couldn't squeeze her hand back, she began crying more. I tried to comfort her, but my speech was a mess.

I felt horrible that my children had to witness this happening. My 10-year-old son was crying while my 12-year-old daughter was pacing back and forth next to the car, also crying. Of course, my wife was trying to keep our children calm and keep herself together at the same time. To this day, I still don't know how she managed to accomplish both. All I knew was that it was the scariest thing I'd ever been through in my entire life. All I could picture was being permanently crippled and paralyzed on one side of my body as I worried about what this would do to my family.

A few minutes later, the paramedics showed up and started evaluating me. I have to tell you that I've never had an issue with high blood pressure, a trait that I picked up from my father who was always well over 300 pounds, never exercised and consumed the Standard American diet until the day he died like it was going out of style. My blood pressure typically stays right around 110/78, but at that moment it was 172/119. Even though I had a massive headache I was relieved that my right arm was slowly starting to get a little bit of feeling back in it. The paramedics loaded me up and off to the hospital we went.

Over the next hour as I laid waiting in the emergency room, my headache started subsiding and I slowly regained the feeling in my right side, which, as you can imagine, was a massive relief to me and my wife. I was so worried I would suffer permanent paralysis, but I was lucky.

I had to stay in the hospital overnight as they ran an entire series of tests from bloodwork to an EKG, ultrasound of the carotid arteries in my neck, MRI, X-rays and a CAT scan, all of which turned up absolutely nothing as an explanation of what had happened to me. Their final diagnosis was that I had suffered a TIA, or Transient Ischemic Attack (also called a mini-stroke). It still involves a temporary loss of blood flow to a part of the brain, but fortunately, the effects are usually not long-term.

The doctor did warn me, however, that people who suffer a TIA are at an increased risk of having another one within the next 12 months. Ironically, about 5 months prior to this event, I had started a new eating plan, cleaned up my eating all the way around and had already lost about 40 pounds by the time I experienced the TIA. The doctor told me that if I hadn't done that, the end result would have probably been much worse. I have always been grateful for changing my outlook on food when I did.

How does all of this tie into low cholesterol? Ironically, when I was checked into the hospital, my cholesterol was 105. It had never been above 160- even when I was eating junk every day and not taking care of myself- including a complete absence of exercise. When my functional medicine doctor saw my low cholesterol rate, she immediately put me on a plan to bring the number up. She realized just how important it was.

But proof of the importance of maintaining a healthy cholesterol doesn't stop there. As I mentioned earlier, having low cholesterol damages the brain. In a recent study, scientists from the Davis Alzheimer's Disease Research Center found that older individuals who had higher levels of LDL, or "bad" cholesterol and lower levels of HDL, or "good" cholesterol, had a significantly higher risk of developing Alzheimer's. By the way, calling LDL "bad" cholesterol is actually an unwarranted title since the purpose for us having LDL in the first place is to ensure that cholesterol makes it to the cells throughout our body. This is yet another way that we have been wrong about cholesterol all these years.

While the base root of what causes Alzheimer's is still unknown, researchers know that one contributing factor lies in a substance known as amyloid plaque, which just so happens to be the exact same plaque that causes a buildup in your heart. When HDL is low and LDL is high (which is usually the scenario), it allows the brain to build up levels of a protein called beta-amyloid. Whenever this protein is allowed to collect in the brain, the risk of contracting Alzheimer's increases substantially- especially since the health of the brain is already jeopardized by the death of neurons due to Parkinson's disease.

There's more viable evidence that we've been on the wrong track. In another recent study conducted at the Mayo Clinic, they found that individuals who consumed the highest amounts of saturated fats showed a 44 percent *decrease* in the risk of developing dementia. That doesn't mean that you can throw caution to the wind and eat a plate full of fat at every meal, but it does say that individuals who refrain from restricting fat in their diets are at a significantly lower risk of developing dementia later in their lives.

The same study compared individuals who predominantly chose a much higher ratio of carbs over fat to those who consumed the most fat and found that the carb group's risk of dementia shot up an unbelievable 89 percent.

Another study performed around the same time shows that including high amounts of saturated fats in your diet had no increased risk of cardiovascular issues, further grounding the fact that saturated fats are the basis of healthy brain cells. It should come as no shock that one of the most abundant sources of saturated fat can be found in a woman's breast milk.

An additional study, whose results were published in the journal Neurology, which is the official journal of The American Academy of Neurology, showed that those among the elderly with the highest cholesterol levels could expect a decreased risk of dementia by as much as 70 percent.

If you need one last piece of proof that cholesterol is good for you, take it straight from the mouth of the Food and Drug Administration (FDA). They have become so convinced about the importance of maintaining proper cholesterol levels that they've taken their own steps to get the word out. So strong is their conviction on the matter that in 2012, they started issuing consumer warnings about the dangers of specific prescription medications whose intended use was to lower cholesterol, basing their actions on the studies that clearly show a link between low cholesterol and an increase of memory decline and other brain issues. You don't have to take my word for it: the results of these actions are available online by doing a simple search.

But let's back up a minute. None of this evidence is supposed to tout

LDL cholesterol as being harmless. Like many other compounds, it can cause you harm when it is misused. That's where the harmful effects of sugar once again comes into play. When excess sugar is present in your body, it attaches to LDL cholesterol and becomes oxidized through a process known as glycation. Once it becomes oxidized, it turns it into a health risk.

Since I was an admitted sugaraholic, I needed to make some drastic changes to my eating plan. Actually, that's not an accurate statement because I didn't really have a plan. I ate as much as I wanted of whatever I wanted, whenever I wanted it. *That* was my plan. But I soon found out that food is very important when it comes to Parkinson's, which brings me to the next thing I wish I'd known when I was first diagnosed:

Insight #7: The Importance of Eating Balanced Meals

I've known all my life that I was supposed to eat healthy foods, but when you're a kid you don't know any better and you certainly don't care enough to be concerned. As a teenager, you think you're invincible because you have your entire life ahead of you and you're about to set free into the world. As a young adult, you decide you'll worry about it when you get older because, at the time, you have too many things that are more important to worry about. And when you develop Parkinson's, you look back and wish that you had spent all those years taking better care of yourself.

We all know we're supposed to eat nutritious, balanced meals, but that still isn't always a good enough incentive for some of us to actually do it on a regular basis. We need more motivation than that. So how about this? Do it to help your Parkinson's.

Unfortunately, there is no specific or perfect eating plan recommended for Parkinson patients so you are left having to rely on yourself to make the right decisions when it comes to food. We are encouraged to remember that proper nutrition is one of the best things you can do to help manage your disease.

At the time that I was diagnosed, I weighed around 230, having already lost 30 pounds on my clean eating plan. Although I still had a good bit of weight to go to get down to my goal, I felt amazing compared to how I felt before. That's because I had discovered what was making me feel so horrible.

I wasn't stupid: I knew that all the fast food I had been inhaling was the reason I had weighed 260 pounds on a 5 foot 11 inch frame, but carrying around all that excess weight wasn't motivation enough as long as they still made shorts with elastic in the waist. I had to have the truth (and by that I mean Parkinson's) slap me in the face in order to get my full attention. It's sad that it took such an extreme measure to wake me up.

Right after I was diagnosed, my wife had started seeing a functional medicine doctor in our area who specialized in treating the causes of disease instead of just throwing medicine at them (what a noble concept). My wife had been diagnosed with Celiac disease and had been placed on a special regimen that not only helped her heal her gut, but a positive side effect was that she lost 62 pounds and had completely eliminated her heart palpitations. My wife encouraged me to see if this doctor could help me with my Parkinson's so based on those kinds of results, I took a chance and went to see her. It literally changed my life.

She ran a full blood panel on me, looking for specific markers that could be contributing to my disease. When the results came in, I was beyond shocked. That brings us to the next chapter where I talk about my next thing I wish I had known when I was first diagnosed:

Insight #8: The Importance of Food Sensitivity and Gluten Testing

Chapter 8

Food Sensitivity And The Role It Plays In Your Health

You have no idea how important the information I'm about to share with you is to your health. Let's just put it this way: it saved my life and the life of my wife. That's no exaggeration. The scary part was that while my wife had obvious symptoms that something was wrong, I didn't. I had no idea what was going on in my body. Oh sure, I knew I was overweight because I was eating junk, but anyone could have come to that conclusion. It wasn't exactly a revelation. But it never occurred to me that the food I was eating was what was actually making me sick.

Food sensitivity is one of the most common issues facing us today, but it's also one of the most overlooked. Traditional doctors prefer to prescribe medication for symptoms instead of getting to the root of things and looking at what's causing the symptoms in the first place. They don't do this on purpose and they aren't purposely trying to keep us sick. They do it because in all of their studies and in all of their training, they are never taught about the importance of proper nutrition and how much it impacts your health. How sad that is.

Doctors are trained to look for symptoms and to match those symptoms with the proper diagnosis, which they do quite well, but never once are they trained to look to food for the answers.

Think about the last few times you've gone to the doctor about a medical issue other than Parkinson's. Did your doctor ever bring up the subject of what you were eating? Did they suggest that at least some, if not all, of your symptoms could be somehow related to food? Did they advise you to eliminate or add specific foods into your eating plan? I'd be willing to bet there's a good chance you answered "no" to these questions. Again, this isn't their fault. This is how they were trained.

If you're overweight they can instruct you to eat healthier, but their direction never goes any farther than that. It always reverts back to focusing on the symptoms, over and over again. This is the wrong approach.

Symptoms of Food Sensitivity

Healing food sensitivities requires taking the proper steps. Unless you remove the foods that you are sensitive to from your diet, you can't possibly expect to ever recover and heal. You'll keep contaminating yourself over and over again and you'll end up chasing your tail and never getting better. You have to start with elimination and move forward from there. But you can't remove the offending foods unless you know which ones are causing problems and you can't know that unless you are able to identify food sensitivity symptoms.

Ask anyone their idea of what food sensitivity would look like and the first thing that comes to mind is probably an upset stomach or diarrhea. We have this preconceived notion that the best way our body can tell us that it doesn't agree with something we eat is through digestive issues. But that's just a small piece of the puzzle. Food sensitivity can manifest in many other ways- hidden ways that you would never know to make the connection with.

Oftentimes, a Parkinson patient (or anyone, for that matter) will have a sensitivity to a particular food and not realize it because they eat that food all the time so their body never gets over the current bout of sensitivity before they once again introduce that food back into their system.

An individual could be experiencing diarrhea, gas, bloating, cramping and reflux and never put two-and-two together. They accept their digestive issues as being "the norm", convince themselves that it's just the price they have to pay (and are willing to pay) for enjoying all of their favorite foods and never give it a second thought. But anytime you body reacts in this manner to you eating something, it's trying to tell you something. It's saying, "Hey! I don't like that! And this is how I'm going to show my displeasure!'"

So what are the symptoms of having a food sensitivity?

1. Cravings. Do you have a particular food that you feel you just can't live without? You've tried giving it up in the past and were met with disastrous results each and every time you've tried to deny yourself of this pleasure. Or are you willing to clean up all areas of your eating *except* for that one food? Well, guess what? Like it or not, you probably have a sensitivity to it.

Having a food craving means that moderation goes out the window wherever this food is concerned. There's no such thing as "a little bit won't hurt anything" because all it takes is a little bit to elicit a reaction. You tend to amplify those disastrous results by overindulging.

It might seem a bit counterintuitive for your body to crave something that makes it ill, but that's the way it works, nonetheless. Here's how that scenario plays out: you eat something that you're sensitive to. Because of you body's reaction it isn't able to digest it properly so instead of it being processed and distributed through your system like other foods, it sits in your gut, literally rotting while your body tries to decide what to do with it. It's presence there causes irritation which eventually creates little fissures, or holes, in your gut lining, allowing the undigested particles of food to then leak out into your system. Your body recognizes that something is there that shouldn't be and its immune response is to send antibodies to deal with the intruder in the same way that it would handle any other foreign body.

Unfortunately for you, you body doesn't realize that this is a single attack on its system so it produces a preemptive strike and disperses additional antibodies as a wave of protection from possible future attacks. But with the threat neutralized and nothing left to attack, the antibodies are left hanging around without a purpose. Since they have nothing to do, they want to be put to good use so they begin craving something that will require their assistance. Their craving now becomes your craving.

2. Skin issues. Anytime you eat something that you shouldn't your body's negative response is going to show up in your skin. We see many examples of this all the time, but never know the real reason behind them. Dark circles under the eyes, puffy and glassy eyes, acne, rosacea, rashes, a ruddy complexion, rough, dry skin and itchy skin are all signs of toxins brewing in your body. Remember that you skin is the largest organ of your body so it makes sense that it would show signs that something's not right.

3. Joint pain. That painful shoulder that you thought was just due to arthritis or sleeping on one side too much probably has nothing to do with either. Chances are its inflammation flaring up in your joints- the most profound area at the moment being your shoulder.

Reflux, heartburn and GERD. Many people get heartburn, which is caused by your stomach acid backing up into your esophagus. But why does your stomach acid do that? While it could be due to your lower esophageal sphincter muscle not restricting properly, it's usually caused by the foods that we eat. Spicy foods can do the trick, but so can foods that we're sensitive to.

Reflux and GERD, or gastro esophageal reflux disease, doesn't just happen on its own. It isn't random and it isn't an accident. There has to be a specific reason behind it. There is always an underlying issue that causes your stomach acid to churn itself up and go to the effort of defying gravity and pumping itself back up into your esophagus.

5. Brain fog. Ever had "fuzzy thinking"? Ever felt like you were having trouble concentrating and focusing on things? Have you had bouts where your brain didn't seem to be functioning up to par more than the usual? These are all signs that your brain is experiencing a morphine-like satisfaction for specific foods that you're hypersensitive to, caused by natural compounds from the opium plant family called casomorphins and gluteomorphins. These compounds register in the same part of the brain that you would receive pleasure from morphine or other similar mind-altering

compounds.

6. Fatigue. Eating foods that are good for you are digested and turned into energy that your body utilizes to run off of. Eating foods that you are sensitive to means they can't be utilized by the body and are thus turned into inflammation, which triggers an immune response. These two reactions zap your energy and make you feel sluggish and sick, plus you feel that way because you're also being denied the nutrients and vitamins that would make you feel healthy and energetic.

7. Constipation. How often do you have a bowel movement? If you've been diagnosed with Parkinson's you already know what a challenge it can be to stay regular. If you haven't been diagnosed you can still have these same challenges because of a food sensitivity and they will produce the same results as they do to someone with Parkinson's.

But besides the aggravation of not being able to go to the bathroom on a regular basis, cramping, bloating and the general overall uncomfortable feeling that it creates, you also have to be concerned about your medication because when you're gut isn't functioning properly, your meds aren't being absorbed into your body and you won't get the full effects from them. Many times, a person with undiscovered food sensitivities will start to believe that their medications are no longer effective when, in actuality, they aren't getting the chance to do what they were designed to do because they're not being properly absorbed into your system.

Gluten

Chances are you've probably heard of gluten at some point, maybe even in passing while talking to a friend, but unless you've been told you have an issue with it you probably don't know a whole lot about it, which is completely understandable. But gluten is something that everyone should be aware of because it poses a massive threat to all of us. That's right, I said ALL of us.

Most people don't give gluten a second thought unless they find out they're allergic to it and then it suddenly becomes a life-altering issue- and for good reason. It's like being told you have an allergy to peanuts or bee stings. Once you've been told that you have such a severe allergy to something and you have a clear understanding of just how serious that allergy is, you'll go out of your way to stay as far away from these things as you can. We should all incorporate that same level of thinking to gluten.

When I had my testing, I was lucky that I didn't have many sensitivities to foods. But I did have a big problem that needed my immediate attention because I found out that I was allergic to gluten.

Although gluten has been around for many years, it has received a tremendous amount of exposure just during the last few years with the vast majority of it being negative. So what's all the fuss about? Why has this compound become such a concern for so many people? By the way, most people have no idea what gluten is even though they've heard the term used. But given the medical complications that it creates, it's certainly worth taking the time to research it so you know what you're up against. Plus, it has to do with what gluten is doing to our health as a whole that warrants your attention.

Gluten is a protein composite that is found in wheat and other grains. It's what gives these products their elasticity and keeps them bound together (gluten in Latin means "glue"), helps them retain their shape and gives them a chewy consistency.

Gluten sensitivity isn't a rare condition. Approximately 80 percent of the population has a sensitivity to gluten. As I stated before, none of us were designed to process gluten. The only reason some of us don't show obvious signs of getting sick from it is because our guts have managed to develop antibodies, which keep it at bay. But that doesn't mean that it isn't still causing you some kind of issues that you haven't yet connected to gluten. Theoretically, you could go your entire life and have minor issues that you never connect to a gluten sensitivity.

Gluten is a much bigger issue than most people realize. Only a few years ago, you would have seen very few items in your grocery store or sold online that were "gluten free". Many dismissed it as nothing more than the latest diet fad. Now, those products are everywhere. The list of manufacturers who are trying to meet these growing needs is constantly growing, as are the list of available products. And you can expect the list of foods to continue on this growth because more and more people are finding out just how damaging gluten is for them.

Now, this might come as a shock to you, but it should be mentioned that grains, in general, are not good for us, anyway. Nature actually designed grains with their own built-in defense mechanism called lectins. But these aren't the same kind of lectins found in so many different foods. Those lectins are fine to consume. The lectins found in grains, however, are something totally different because they are proteins that our bodies are not designed to digest.

Here's how it works. When you eat protein, your body digests it, turns it into amino acids before being picked up and absorbed by the small intestines. But the lectins found in grains are vastly different. They were naturally placed in grains as a deterrent to keep pests from eating them. Insects eat the grains, the lectins attack their digestive system and the insects decide it isn't worth the discomfort they're experiencing and they move on to something else that doesn't put up such a fight.

Now man comes along and decides it would be a good idea to eat grains. Never mind that the same detrimental lectins that were a deterrent for insects are still present. Instead of heeding the warning that nature has put in place, we decide to throw caution to the wind, disregard that warning and eat to our heart's content. The result? Grains make us sick.

First, you have to look at the fact that wheat (gluten) actually restricts the amount of blood flow into the brain's frontal cortex. That can't be good, right? But this isn't some new revelation. It's been documented in studies dating all the way back to the early 1950s.

One of the most recent of these studies occurred in 1997 and was published in the "Journal of Internal Medicine", involved a brain scan which showed an obvious restriction in blood flow of a patient with "schizophrenic disorder". After the patient was placed on a gluten-free diet, not only did blood flow to the brain normalize, but the patient's intestinal issues were eliminated and their condition disappeared.

In 2004, another study revealed that consuming gluten caused "cerebral hypoperfusion", or a decrease in blood flow to the brain. This study, conducted by a collaboration of researchers from the Institute of Internal Medicine, Catholic University, Rome, Italy, involved a larger group of participants with celiac disease, depression and anxiety. When gluten was eliminated, their conditions improved dramatically.

But to get the full scope of what is being said here, you have to fully open your mind to what cerebral hypoperfusion means. When you restrict blood flow to an organ, you're limiting that organ's capabilities, jeopardizing its health and, dare we say, threatening its very existence. That's bad enough news if you're a kidney or the liver. But just imagine if you're talking about the brain: the hub of your central nervous system: the organ that facilities your thinking, reasoning, memory, cognitive skills, learning capabilities and, in the instances of Parkinson's patients, your very movements, themselves. Now, you're talking serous issues.

We now know that grains not only damage the brain, but they also cause cataclysmic repercussions. It not only disrupts the way neurons deal with glucose, but it lowers their ability to function and, in some instances, when the sensitivity is severe enough, it *kills* them.

But don't just take my word for it. If you don't think gluten can be a major contributor to many of the medical issues plaguing us today, consider the fact that gluten's negative impact on our health has been journaled in, of all places, Medline, which is the biomedical database for the National Library of Medicine. Medline currently has approximately 10,000 references to gluten, with the list continuously growing exponentially. If *they* recognize it as a health concern, it certainly deserves *our* attention, as well, don't you agree?

We've talked about how gluten can affect our brain so now let's look at the damage from a digestive point-of-view. When you eat grains, the lectins prevent the proteins found in them from being absorbed. Instead, they pass through the gut unprocessed. Once they reach your intestines, this undigested mass of protein begins to irritate the lining of the intestines until small holes appear. The undigested proteins pass out into your blood stream where they're carried all over the body to all the places they aren't supposed to be.

Wait, it gets worse. You now have undigested proteins working their way into all the nooks and crannies of your body. Your body senses the presence of a foreign matter and commands your immune system to send antibodies to attack the invader and dispose of it. Since your immune system is already highly sensitive to your gut, it takes immediate and severe action (it does this because your gut is such an important part of your overall health).

Here in lies the problem. These harmful lectins that have maneuvered their way throughout your body often resemble your own tissue. That means that when your immune system begins attacking everything that it perceives to be a threat, it can't differentiate between the two and your own tissue gets mistakenly thrown into the mix. The result? Inflammation.

The reason your body mistakenly attacks it's own self is because of a case of mistaken identity. The main protein found in gluten, gliadin, closely resembles many of the tissues found in the human body-specifically those of some of our organs, such as the pancreas, putting it at risk.

But that's *still* not the worst part. Some of the tissue that your immune system attacks isn't just ordinary tissue: it's organs. Now that they've been placed under attack, this causes the organs to run inefficiency, which, of course, causes various symptoms to begin to appear. This raises all kinds of medical issues for you out of nowhere and begins to make you sick. You go to the doctor and they prescribe medication for your symptoms when, in reality, your body is attacking it's own organs because of inflammation brought on by gluten. Of course, this condition has a name: it's called autoimmune disease. Pretty amazing, huh?

How do I know this? Because my wife and I were living it.

My wife had so much inflammation in her body from gluten and some other things (I'll cover those in a moment) that her gut was making her sick every day. She was experiencing all kinds of digestive issues and her food wasn't digesting. It couldn't because her gut had suffered too much damage. This meant that she wasn't processing or absorbing hardly any of her vitamins and nutrients. Even if she were to eat a salad with steamed vegetables, she would only receive a minuscule amount of the benefits from it. Everything made her sick. *Everything.* How would you like to wake up every single day of your life knowing that whatever you ate was going to make you sick? Not very encouraging, is it? That was her world.

So how did she still manage to gain weight? Because by some sick twist of irony, it seems that fat and calories still manage to find their way through and take up residence in your body, even though you don't get the benefit of any of the good stuff.

My wife was placed on a repair diet (I use the word "diet" loosely since it was actually the proper way of eating that we should have been on all along), she healed her gut and lost 62 pounds. She also eliminated her heart palpitations (which were completely ruining her life) and finally felt fantastic after many years of feeling like crap. Her skin looked smoother, her hair was shinier, her face had a glow to it and she was noticeably happier all the way around. All because she eliminated gluten from her diet. I'm so proud of her.

When I said I would cover the other things that she was forced to eliminate from her diet I was talking about the other things that were unknowingly making her sick. Through testing we found out that these items were corn, soy and dairy. These were also causing her to have a reaction, although it was nowhere near the intensity as gluten was causing.

If she was told to avoid gluten, corn, soy and dairy, you're probably wondering what that left her to eat, right? Well, she ate everything that we were supposed to be eating, but weren't. You see, we all think we can fool our bodies. We might have eaten everything we wanted when we were young and never worried about it because we never saw any repercussions from it. But the sad part is that it always catches up with you. Maybe not now and maybe not within the next year or so, but eventually, it *will* catch up to you and when it does, you'll have to contend with your own set of health issues all because of food sensitivities, such as gluten.

That was my wife's story: now let me tell you mine (you're going to love this).

At the beginning of this post, I said I didn't have any real food sensitivities except for gluten. I do need to reiterate that I have a small sensitivity to dairy, which I try to avoid anyway since I'm lactose-intolerant, but it isn't a life-changer for me if I have dairy in small amounts. But just having that one major food sensitivity of gluten made up for everything.

One of the tests that you should have (in fact, it's so important that EVERYONE should have this test), is called the IgG food allergy test (you'll hear this name again), which stands for Immunoglobulin G. It's purpose is to determine the amount of sensitivity your body responds to from certain foods. Of course, the higher a food rates, the more sensitive you are to that food.

When an individual eats something that they are sensitive to, the body's immune system responds by releasing histamine, an organic compound. Histamine is our natural way of dealing with an allergen, such as pollen, an insect bite or, in this case, a specific food.

But there is one major difference between an allergic reaction to pollen and one from foods. When you suffer a reaction from pollen, the reaction is instantaneous. But when it involves food, the reaction could be delayed hours or even up to three days. This makes it virtually impossible to distinguish which foods are making you sick.

That's why the IgG test is necessary. It tests a total of 93 different foods to determine which ones are causing you problems and how much of a threat they are to your health. Once they're identified, you can remove them from your diet and begin healing from the inside out.

When my results came back for gluten, my doctor was speechless. She had never seen numbers like mine before. The range for gluten sensitivity is measure using a scale between a 1 and a 6, with 1 meaning an individual has a slight allergic reaction to gluten and a 6 meaning they have a severe reaction to gluten.

Mine was 17.

You read that right. My allergic reaction rated almost *three* times the highest point on the scale. That explained why I was so sick and always felt so crummy.

Now, you need to know that gluten affects different people in different ways. Through my wife's IgG testing, we discovered that she was also allergic to gluten and that her sensitivity manifested itself as heart palpitations. Once she eliminated gluten from her diet, the palpitations completely went away. But gluten affected me in a very different way. It was attacking my brain.

I'll never forget what my functional medicine doctor told me. She looked at me and said: "gluten is literally shredding your brain." Believe me: if that doesn't get you on the path to eliminating gluten, nothing will. I haven't had gluten since.

In my case, gluten was causing inflammation in my brain just like my wife's inflammation was damaging her heart. This certainly wasn't something a Parkinson patient wants to hear, but, at the same time, I needed to hear it.

As I weaned off of gluten, I began to realize that gluten had been amplifying my symptoms. Even worse, it was accelerating the progression of the disease due to the fact that it was attacking my brain. The only way I could ever tell if I had been exposed was my stomach would become upset. So that became the guideline that I used since my brain had no way of warning me.

I have to be careful when I eat, but it's well worth the effort not have to worry about what it's doing to me. When my wife and I go out, we can only go to certain places. We have to give specific instructions to how our food is prepared and even then, we occasionally get "glutened". While it isn't a fool-proof plan it's still a far cry from the amount of gluten we were ingesting on a daily basis. The good news is that more restaurants are offering gluten-free menus to accommodate the growing number of people who can't have gluten.

If you have testing preformed and you find out that you have a gluten allergy, you'll have to stay on your toes when it comes to eating at someone's house. Most people don't have a clue about gluten, what it does or how dangerous it can be so you'll have to be proactive about protecting yourself. Others won't intentionally try to cause you harm, but they'll unknowingly do it just because they won't know any better.

How will you know if you've been glutened? If your reaction is shown as a physical symptom, such as heart palpitations, for example, your body will be more than happy to tell you when you've been exposed. On the other hand, if your symptoms only target your brain, it makes it a little tougher so you'll just have to be extra careful.

How Gluten Affects The Brain

I don't want you to think that my negative experience with gluten is an isolated incident. There's tons of concrete evidence that supports the fact that gluten damages the brain. Some of the most renowned doctors in the country are onboard with the crusade to warn the general public about just how dangerous gluten can be. In fact, there's even a medical term for it called "gluten-sensitive idiopathic neuropathy".

The most common neurological condition caused by a gluten sensitivity is cerebellar ataxia. This condition causes irreparable damage to the cerebellum. While it can be caused by injury or as a result of prolonged exposure to nicotine or alcohol it is more commonly caused by a sensitivity to gluten. When gluten is the culprit, the condition is appropriately called gluten ataxia.

This is how gluten ataxia works: when you eat gluten, your body responds by producing antibodies in an attempt to fight off the invader, initially causing inflammation and resulting in damage later on. But in the process of attacking, these antibodies also attack the cerebellum, the part of your brain that deals with such things as motor control, coordination, balance and muscle control. Ironically, even though gluten is the reason for the attack, it isn't the gluten that is causing the damage to your brain but rather your own white cells responding to the presence of the foreign matter, which in this case is gluten. Once the brain is affected in this manner the damage is irreversible.

For those with Parkinson's, symptoms of gluten ataxia can start out small and remain relatively unnoticed. It typically begins as a mild difficulty with balance and progresses into a slight difficulty in walking. Normal, smooth actions will become more difficult as you begin to lose your coordination. As time goes on and symptoms worsen, the individual will see a decrease in their fine motor skills, making it more difficult to control their handwriting and even their speech. Since these symptoms so closely correlate with those of Parkinson's disease, you can see why they can be blamed on Parkinson's, allowing for the detection of gluten ataxia to be so easily overlooked and opening the door for the condition to worsen.

The problem with identifying gluten ataxia is that it is a relatively newly-identified condition, leaving some doctors still in the learning phase about it. But considering the risk that you're taking by not taking action, it's worth bringing it to their attention and discussing with your doctor so you can undergo testing to rule it out. With this disease, time is of the essence since 60 percent of those who have it experience cerebellar atrophy, or brain shrinkage.

Another problem facing patents is that many of our doctors aren't accepting of the fact that our brains and our guts are somehow linked together. They typically treat one or the other separately without giving a second thought to the possibility that one disorder might be directly associated with the other. Why is there such a strong link between the gut and the brain? Because the two *are* connected.

Did you know that 70 percent of your body's immune cells are located in the digestive system? This is no accident. Think about the fact that when you're nervous, you get "butterflies", when you're upset your stomach churns and when you're angry it knots up. These are not coincidences. This is your gut's "brain" talking to you. The "brain" located in your gut that is responsible for this and so many other responses from your body is called the enteric nervous system. And this is precisely why gluten landing in your gut can end up having such a massive impact on your brain.

Instead of your emotions always determining your physical state of health (such as worrying making you nauseous), there is just as much influence the other way. Having digestive issues (such as from a gluten sensitivity) can play a major role in your emotional and psychological well-being. My case is a prime example of that. I had no obvious digestive issues with gluten but, at the same time, it was slowly destroying my brain.

Even though we've talked about how having a gluten sensitivity can directly impact your brain, your brain isn't where the gluten ends up. It ends up in your gut because you've eaten it. If there wasn't a neurological connection between the gut and the brain you wouldn't be affected, you'd just have an upset stomach. If you want further proof, think about the fact that people with digestive issues are more likely to suffer from depression or anxiety than people who don't.

Chapter 9

What You Should Know About Inflammation

Even though I mentioned inflammation earlier, I've only briefly touched on the subject. Since inflammation is such a massive problem in so many people's lives I decided it needed an entire chapter all to itself. But even with this being such a major health issue in our society- on so many levels- that still isn't the real reason why we should be concerned about inflammation. We should be concerned because so many people aren't aware of just how widespread and dangerous of an issue it really is.

I'm going to talk about inflammation and who it is connected to food. Once we've ingested a food that we are sensitive to, the body begins to suffer from inflammation, which is the catalyst for many of the health issues that we experience today and why it's important that everyone be able to recognize all the sneaky ways that inflammation can show itself.

At some point in our lives every one of us has experienced inflammation in one form or another. Outwardly, it could be seen in action as a result of a cut or a burn. Inwardly, it occurs when a joint suffers injury. But although you've heard about how inflammation is a natural occurrence of the body and how important it is for proper healing to take place, chances are you don't know the full story as to how it relates to Parkinson's.

From a positive standpoint, inflammation is a necessary part of the healing process that our bodies go through when it becomes damaged. It is our body's first step in healing itself when we suffer damage. Whether it's an external injury, an internal injury, a prolonged illness or merely stress, inflammation plays a key role in bringing our body back to health. In these instances, inflammation is a good thing. It's when inflammation isn't supposed to be present that things can turn ugly- really fast.

Inflammation is only meant to be a temporary solution to a problem. If you cut yourself, your body is designed to immediately go to work to repair the site and supply it with what it needs to bring it back to health. In the meantime, you'll experience swelling, redness and tenderness as the body goes through the repair stages. As soon as treatment is completed, inflammation is meant to go away.

When inflammation isn't serving a purpose of healing, it can be disastrous to your health because it can appear in so many disguises. In fact, you probably aren't aware of just how common inflammation is or how many different ways it can show up. According to statistics from the medical community, out of the top ten causes of death in the U.S., inflammation is connected to seven of them:

- Alzheimer's disease
- cancer
- chronic lower respiratory disease
- type 2 diabetes
- heart disease
- nephritis, or inflammation of the kidneys
- stroke

Inflammation is caused by many different things, but they all conveniently fall into either one of two categories: food and stress. We'll talk about stress in Chapter 10.

From a food standpoint, inflammation occurs either because of

(1) the harmful foods that we eat
 and/or
(2) the amount of harmful foods that we eat.

Nowadays, when you consider the Standard American Diet consisting of fast food, junk food, processed, canned, frozen, instant or microwaveable products, you're talking about both the choice and the amount. Instead of just abusing our bodies by making harmful food choices, we abuse it twice by not only consuming these harmful foods, but by consuming massive quantities of them. There is no conceivable way you can hope to escape inflammation by following that kind of a botched plan- no matter how healthy you are. It simply can't be done. You're destined to fail before you even get started.

Some types of harmful foods which encourage inflammation are:

- Animal fats. Unless otherwise specified as being grass-fed, today's meat is barn-raised under deplorable conditions. Animals are contained indoors without fresh air and sunshine where they can't roam around foraging and building muscle (giving meat a higher fat content) and must be fed antibiotics to ward off disease from living in their own filth in such close quarters. They're also given growth hormones to speed maturity so they can be brought to market faster. Even the grains that they are fed are genetically-modified organisms (GMOs), meaning that their DNA has been altered in a lab. All of these features are passed on into the meats that we consume.

- Hydrogenated and Partially-hydrogenated fats. These are harmful fats, which promote damage to our cells.

- Processed meats. These are any kind of pickled or processed meats (bologna, salami, pepperoni, for example). They contain artificial coloring, artificial flavorings, additives and preservatives, none of which are natural and all of which are not healthy for us to consume.

- Sugar (all 50-plus derivatives of it).

Acute Versus Chronic

There are two types of inflammation: acute and chronic. Acute inflammation kicks into action, say, from when you cut your finger. The body senses an injury and deploys white blood cells to the area to start the healing process. Acute inflammation is a necessary function of the body and only lasts until the injury has sufficiently healed.

There are two parts to acute inflammation: (1) attacking the issue that has caused damage to the body (a cut, burn or joint pain) while trying to lower the risk of infection as much as possible, and (2) repairing said damage through the use of the immune system by growing healthy cells to make new tissue. In a perfect scenario, inflammation works as it is supposed to and the body recovers. But there are times when inflammation happens when it isn't needed. This spells bad news for the individual. This is when you experience chronic inflammation.

How common is chronic inflammation? Statistically, one in every ten people have some form of chronic inflammation with women being nine times as likely to develop it as men. The thing you need to remember about chronic inflammation is that it serves as a warning. It's your body warning you that something isn't right. And this particular type of warning is like standing on the tracks with an oncoming train barreling towards you. It isn't going to go away on it's own, the situation is only going to get worse and the only way you're going to be safe again is to find a way to put a stop to it.

The first part of chronic inflammation is when the body starts to attack the issue causing the disruption, which in this case is the food that you eat. Your body is smart enough to recognize when something shouldn't be there because of the potential health threat that it poses. So it speaks to you in the only way it can- with symptoms. Here are just a few of the common symptoms of chronic inflammation, some of which I'm sure you'll be surprised to see:

- acid reflux (heartburn)
- Alzheimer's disease
- asthma
- atherosclerosis
- bronchitis
- cancer
- chronic Hepatitis- active
- cirrhosis
- Crohn's disease
- dementia

- dermatitis
- diverticulitis
- eczema
- edema
- fibromyalgia
- hypertension
- Irritabel Bowel Syndrome
- lupus
- peptic ulcer- chronic
- periodontitis- chronic
- rheumatoid arthritis
- scleroderma- connective tissue disease
- sinusitis
- spastic colon
- tendonitis
- tuberculosis
- ulcerative colitis

As it relates to food, chronic inflammation is brought on in one of three ways (or, sometimes, even a combination, thereof): (1) making poor food choices, (2) an excessive caloric intake and (3) elevated blood sugar levels. Here is an explanation of each:

(1) Poor food choices. When you choose foods that your body is sensitive to (whether you're aware of it or not), the food elicits an allergic response in your gut. In return, the body's immune system releases it's own protective measures, macrophages and mast cells, to counteract this intrusion. The war that rages between these two forces causes damage to the lining of you gut, making it much easier for food to pass through and out into the bloodstream.

(2) Excessive calorie intake. Despite popular belief, you do not add fat cells when you gain weight. Your body already contains a certain number of fat cells that you were born with and that stay with you for life. When you put on weight, these fat cells begin to fill with excess fat and swell, adding to the size of your body. At a certain point, they can become too enlarged and start to leak, spilling out fat into the bloodstream and triggering inflammation. Once again, macrophages are called in to clean up the mess. But in the process,

they release chemicals to clean up the spill, the same way you would clean up toxic waste. This combination of leaking fat and responsive chemicals leads to inflammation.

The second part of this scenario is that the inflammation interferes with the proper functioning of the hormone, leptin. Leptin is responsible for satiety, or controlling hunger. When the hunger-controlling capabilities of leptin are disrupted, the brain isn't notified that the individual is sufficiently full and the individual overeat, ultimately causing even more inflammation to occur.

(3) Elevated blood sugar levels. A type 2 diabetic is an adult who either doesn't produce enough insulin or their body is unable to adequately utilize what it is given as it should. Besides constantly fighting to balance blood sugar, these individuals also have to contend with the probability that their condition will cause the release of inflammatory chemicals known as cytokines. When you also take into consideration the amount of visceral fat, or abdominal fat, usually found in diabetics, the risk of inflammation goes up even higher.

The main reason that chronic inflammation is so destructive isn't because of what it does to your body but rather because of how much time it is allowed to run unopposed before we realize that it's there. You see, chronic inflammation isn't flamboyant. It doesn't draw attention to itself or go out of its way to make its presence known. Instead, it's sneaky. It hides behind the scenes and waits. And waits. All the while, it's slowly tearing your body apart and jeopardizing your health without sending up any red flags. The longer it remains untreated, the more damage your body is being subjected to.

Chronic inflammation can not only linger undetected for years, it can lie in waiting for decades. All the while, it's slowly chipping away at your health through a sinus infection here, an upset stomach there, or a nagging, achy joint that just never seems to get completely healed despite the fact that you haven't reinjured it. It's all of these individual instances that culminate into one big problem. The sad part is that the average person never sees it coming. They never put all the signs together because they don't know to. Then, one day, they begin to suffer neurological symptoms (like I did) or heart palpitations (like my wife did) and after they're properly tested, it all begins to make sense, but the damage has been done- sometimes irreparable damage.

Detecting Inflammation

There is a two-fold method for identifying chronic inflammation within the body. The first part involves a thorough examination by your doctor. You need to make sure that your doctor is someone who is open to labeling inflammation symptoms for what they are and not dismissing it as something else. Then, they will want to perform some bloodwork to look for specific inflammation markers and combine it with their physical findings to pinpoint the issues. The markers they should focus on are:

Elevated CRP (C-reactive protein). When your body experiences inflammation, the liver goes to work producing this protein. The more inflammation you're experiencing, the higher your CRP number. CRP can only be detected using bloodwork.

Elevated Homocysteine. There are several reasons why your homocysteine level would be elevated. It could be due to a poor diet or one high in animal protein and low in nutrients. Your B vitamins are some of the most important at helping to keep homocysteine levels under control. Caffeine is a culprit, too, so the more you taper off of it, the better off you'll be. Hypothyroidism is yet another indicator that homocysteine levels are out of whack.

Candida Overgrowth

Many doctors don't recognize candida overgrowth as a viable condition because they perform routine tests on patients and nothing abnormal shows up. But what do you tell the countless people who live with the effects of a candida overgrowth every single day? They certainly aren't imagining it. They can testify that something isn't as it should be or else they would have an explanation for what they're experiencing.

What is candida and why should you be concerned about it? Because it could just be what's helping make you sick.

Simply put, candida is a fungus, which, incidentally, is a form of yeast. We all naturally carry a tiny amount of it in our mouths and our intestines to help us absorb and digest the nutrients in the foods that we eat. As long as candida is contained to this small quantity, everything is fine. It's when candida growth is spurred on and becomes unmanageable that trouble ensues. How does candida growth become so out-of-control? There are a number of ways, many of which you're likely guilty of and didn't even know it. What are they?

- a diet high in both carbohydrates and sugar
- a diet high in fermented foods (i.e., pickles, sauerkraut)
- high alcohol consumption
- antibiotics- particularly those used long-term for treating acne or sinus issues
- oral contraception
- steroid inhalers
- hormone pills
- a highly stressful lifestyle

All of these conditions are a perfect breeding ground for candida yeast. But the problem isn't just that your body is cultivating too much yeast but also what that additional amount of yeast is doing to your body.

Since candida is a type of fungus, it thrives very well in the dark, moist recesses of your digestive tract. But, being a fungus also means that, given the right conditions, it grows very rapidly. Any of the above-listed conditions are ideal to do just that.

The increased amount of yeast becomes too much for the gut and begins to tear away at its walls. Once it penetrates this outer layer, it is free to leak out into your bloodstream and be carried throughout the body, a condition aptly named "leaky gut syndrome", which you've probably heard of before.

How do you know if you have a candidate overgrowth? By looking for the typical signs:

- chronic fatigue or a general "run down" feeling (fibromyalgia)
- digestive issues (bloating, gas, constipation, diarrhea)
- strong cravings for sugar and refined carbs
- development of autoimmune diseases (lupus, Hashimoto's thyroiditis, ulcerative colitis, rheumatoid arthritis, scleroderma, multiple sclerosis)
- headaches
- mood swings, irritability
- depression
- anxiety
- brain fog, difficulty concentrating
- poor memory
- muscle aches
- skin conditions (psoriasis, eczema, rashes, hives)
- fungal infections of skin and/or nails (athlete's foot, toenail fungus)
- severe seasonal allergies
- vaginal infections/urinary tract infections (often recurring)
- vaginal/rectal itching

Now you can see the problem. The list of symptoms is so broad and so general that it could qualify for many medical conditions. This is one of the primary reasons why most people never figure out that it's a candida overgrowth until they've experienced the symptoms for quite some time. By the time they pinpoint what the problem is, it's grown into becoming a very big problem.

While having a candida overgrowth can be life-altering by causing some pretty nasty symptoms, it is not fatal. However, there is a form of candida fungal infection that attacks the bloodstream of individuals with a compromised immune system and is carried throughout the body. If left untreated, this variety can be fatal.

If you find yourself facing many of these symptoms, you need to act immediately because the longer you let it go without treatment, the worse the leakage from your gut will be and the longer it will take for it to properly heal.

Testing methods

How can you test to see if you have a candida overgrowth? The most common approach is to do one of these:

- comprehensive stool testing- checks for the kinds and levels of candida
- bloodwork- called IgG, IgA and IgM, which specifically targets candida antibodies
- urine organix dysbiosis- checks for the presence (or an overabundance) of a candida overgrowth called D-arabinitol: also specifies whether the growth is located in the upper gut or the small intestines, which is important for specifying the right course of treatment you'll need.

If you suspect that you might have a candida overgrowth, but you don't want to go to the trouble of going to the doctor, waiting for them to order the testing, taking the tests and waiting for the results, there is one other detection method that you can use at home. It's called the "candida spit test". It might not sound classy, but it gets the job done.

The process is simple: take a full glass of water and spit into it first thing in the morning before you've eaten or brushed your teeth. As soon as you get out of bed is the perfect time. Then, wait a few minutes. If you can see what appear to be "tentacles" growing down towards the bottom of the glass, originating for the spit then there's a very good chance that you have a candida overgrowth. It's not completely foolproof, but it does have a surprisingly high amount of accuracy in confirming a candida overgrowth.

Treatment

The treatment for a candida overgrowth involves a three-part process. Each part needs to be performed to its completion in order for the entire process to work properly and to totally eliminate your candida problem. If you fail to satisfy any one of these three areas, you might as well start all over again because you'll be right back where you started.

Step #1: Get rid of your yeast overgrowth. If you don't start here and do a thorough job of it, the rest doesn't matter because you'll just be spinning your wheels and going nowhere. The way to successfully eliminate all overgrowth is by changing up your eating. This also involves a three-step approach.

The first part of this step is for you to get rid of all sugar. Since yeast feeds off of sugar, sugar is now your enemy. This is generally the hardest thing for people to do because the sensation for sugar is fueled by the candida. You have to be diligent in finding all of the hidden sugar in foods and drinks (such as flour and alcohol, for example). I'll admit that you're going to be challenged to cave and indulge but you have to remain strong for at least a couple of days to allow enough time for the cravings to begin to subside. Once you're past that point and your sweet cravings have been broken, you'll be able to remain sugar-free until the treatment has ended.

Second, you have to drastically cut down your consumption of carbs. That means limiting yourself to no more than 1 cup of complex carbs in a single day (complex carbs are your potatoes, bread and other grains, pasta, beans and even fruit).

Third, is to eliminate all fermented foods. Those who like to indulge in these foods might not like this notion since fermented foods is known for supporting good bacteria. Unfortunately, it also supports the bad ones, too, so it has to be done.

Step #2: Rebuild your good bacteria levels. Taking probiotics is the answer here. The recommended dosage is anywhere between 25-100 billion units per day. Your doctor will be able to advise you on exactly how much you need.

Step #3: Heal your gut. This means introducing healthy foods that are going to not only boost your good bacteria, but also deter bad bacteria from taking over again. Here is a list of some of the best foods to accomplish this:

- greens- all kinds
- cruciferous vegetables (broccoli, cauliflower, cabbage, kale, Brussel sprouts)
- onion
- garlic
- avocado
- apple cider vinegar
- coconut- especially coconut oil
- seeds (flax, chia, hemp)
- herbs (cilantro, parsley, basil, oregano)

You should know that overcoming and eliminating a candida overgrowth is not a sprint, it's a marathon. The entire process of getting your gut back to health could take as much as 3-6 months- depending on how much damage you've caused yourself. One way to help things along is to take a supplement, such as caprylic acid. This causes damage to the walls of the yeast, weakening it and helping to kill it off.

Just as important as knowing what to eat during the repair process is knowing what to refrain from (besides the most obvious ones like sugar and alcohol):

- processed foods
- breads and pasta
- dairy products- the sugar in milk, lactose, actually encourages candida growth
- artificial sweeteners
- all refined grains and flours
- vinegar (except for apple cider)
- peanuts- because of their natural content of mold

The process for overcoming a candida overgrowth might sound like a long time, but the good news is that you'll begin to feel better fairly soon after starting your elimination regimen. Take this as a sign that you're on the right track and use it as encouragement to keep going. Candida didn't just pop up overnight. It requires a reasonable amount of time to get rid of it so hang in there and just keep thinking about how much better you'll feel once it's over.

Chapter 10

Lifestyle Issues That You Need To Be Aware Of

One of the first things that you'll realize after the shock of hearing a diagnosis finally begins to settle in is that you're going to have to make some lifestyle changes if you want to take the most control over your disease. Some of these changes will be relatively easy for most Parkinson patients to accept, but for others, you'll likely want to fight them every step of the way- not because they're wrong for you, but because they're different than what you consider to be the "norm".

No one likes change, but sometimes change is good- and necessary. "If you continue to do what you've been doing, you have to be willing to accept the same results" (a rough translation from motivational speaker Brian Tracy). When you have Parkinson's disease, this philosophy is not acceptable.

When I say lifestyle changes, I'm not referring to things that are totally radical and unobtainable. They have to be fairly easy or at least offer a suitable reward for any sacrifice that you'll have to make or else, as humans, we won't put forth the effort if we don't think the end will justify the means. But even though these things all have a purpose and they make total sense- even if you don't have Parkinson's- they make so much more sense if you do have it.

When you're first diagnosed, you instinctively know that you're going to have to go through some changes- you just aren't fully aware of what those changes are and how much they're going to impact your life and your health. You hope for better health and slowing the progression of the disease down as much as possible, but the truth is, a vast majority of your future lies in your own hands based on the decisions that you make from this point on. Where you end up ten, twenty or thirty years from now all comes down to the choices that you make starting today.

No one can make you eat the right foods. No one can force you to exercise. No one can convince you to avoid all of the situations that trigger the wrong reactions. You have to decide that you want this for yourself. Your decisions today forecast your level of health tomorrow.

Changes are never easy- especially since we're creatures of habit. But in the case of Parkinson's, you don't really have a choice if you want the most out of life. The only way to beat an enemy is to overwhelm them with effort. You just have to fight and keep fighting because, believe me, that's what Parkinson's is going to do.

There are so many lifestyle changes you probably aren't aware of that will directly impact your health- and not just your Parkinson's health, either, but your overall health, too. All of these have been tested and found to be beneficial to a great number of people. This is not hearsay or fluff and it isn't mild speculation. These are actual lifestyle changes that can directly improve your health.

Water

We can survive for weeks without food, but we all know we can't survive without water. It's a basic necessity and the commodity that determines that we survive the shortest amount of time when deprived of it. Yet, we deprive ourselves of it every single day without even giving it a consideration. We all know that we need water in order to sustain life but do you know how much water you're supposed to be drinking? And even if you do, are you consistently following those guidelines? I'll be the first to admit that for my entire adult life I wasn't.

The rule of thumb is that you're supposed to drink half of your body weight in ounces of water every single day. I know that sounds like a lot of water, but it's not just a casual recommendation made by some stuffy lab coats working in a climate-controlled office: it's a real, factual number backed up by science. It's what your body needs in order to maintain proper hydration levels throughout. Of course, if you are working out or performing strenuous activities such as mowing the grass, you have to take this extra loss of fluid through perspiration into consideration and add water accordingly. You should also get in the habit of drinking throughout a workout or taking brief stops in the middle of strenuous activity so your body never has the opportunity to venture too close to dehydration. You also have to take into account any medications that you're taking that might act as diuretics.

Most of the time we rely on our sense of thirst to inform us when it's time for us to get a drink. But this is an unreliable source of detection because by the time your mouth begins to feel the sensation of thirst, which is less than 3 percent hydration, your body has already reached a mild form of dehydration.

Roughly two-thirds of your body is comprised of water with women tending to have a slightly higher percentage of body fat, which, in contrast, allows them to retain more water than men. The water in our bodies is found in three areas:

- our blood
- our cells
- the area surrounding our cells

But it isn't just the amount of water that makes up our bodies that we want to focus on here. It's *where* that water is located that's crucial. Here is a breakdown of how your level of water is distributed:

- Your bones are about 30 percent water.
- Your muscles and kidneys are 80 percent water.
- Your lungs are 83 percent water.
- Your heart is 73 percent water.

You can see that depriving yourself of water is a lot more serious than just being thirsty. You can really cause yourself a great deal of issues simply by not drinking enough to sustain your body. If you stay properly hydrated all of these equally-important areas will take care of themselves. But for Parkinson's patients, it's a little more complicated than that because in our case, it's the brain that deserves the most attention.

Even though our brains and muscles are comprised of approximately 80 percent water it only takes less than 1 percent dehydration before our mental capacities and our muscles start to become affected. *One percent.* This is why whenever you overdo it and you're dehydrated, the first symptoms you feel are weakness and mental fog because these two areas have the most to lose right from the beginning. Research has shown that drinking as little as a single glass of water when you're in mild dehydration can significantly improve your mental capabilities. But *why* does your brain need so much water? That's a good question and it has a very good answer.

Your brain cells thrive on water. It's part of the delicate balance that keeps them in check and working properly. Of all people to deprive themselves of water, Parkinson patients should never be on the list simply because we can't afford to jeopardize our mental clarity any more than necessary.

We also know that when you're dehydrated, it interferes with proper blood flow. When you take a drink, pressure receptors called "baroreceptors" go to work to direct the much-needed liquid to the most sparse, or thirsty, locations. The fact that water helps to promote good blood flow is great news for a Parkinson patient since the brain is connected to 100,000 miles of blood vessels. Since our body is equipped to make adjustments to blood pressure literally at a moment's notice, those who suffer from hypotension, meaning their blood pressure is too low, benefit from water almost as quickly as they can drink it.

Functions of Water In The Body

Water is utilized in one of five ways in the body:

- to help breakdown the foods that we eat so that each part can be utilized where it is needed
- to transport those vitamins and nutrients to our cells
- to regulate our body temperature
- as a lubricant (for joints) and as a shock absorber for the brain, spinal cord and the eyes
- to remove toxins and products that the body can't utilize

through our waste

On the other end of the spectrum, you should also know that you can actually overdo it by drinking too much water, a condition appropriately called water intoxication. Given the filtering capabilities of the kidneys, it would be rather difficult to consume too much water in such a short period of time, but, nevertheless, it is still possible if someone isn't monitoring themselves correctly. This is a good reason why you should monitor your water intake so you can make sure that you're getting a sufficient amount of water, but not too much.

When you happen to consume too much water, you run the risk of developing a condition known as hyponatremia, which means that the sodium in your body has become too saturated with water. The excess water begins to draw sodium from your cells in order to try to balance out the water-to-sodium ratio. Electrolytes attempt to stabilize this imbalance by shifting to and from the cells. At some point, the cells could become so engorged with water that they actually burst.

Forcing your body to work so hard to maintain this entire balancing act is quite dangerous. Not only can it produce irregular heartbeats, but the additional fluid absorbs into brain tissue and puts added pressure on the brain. This can lead to mild symptoms such as groggy behavior, giving the appearance that the individual is intoxicated, to seizures, coma and, in severe cases, even death.

Constipation

As you can see, it's important to always get the right amount of water into our systems every day since it's vital to help with so many things that we take for granted. But while all of these bodily functions seem to operate just fine on auto-pilot, one sometimes requires a little extra help. That one thing that we hold near and dear to our hearts is waste removal.

Anyone with Parkinson's disease will tell you that one of its unfortunate symptoms is constipation. This might not have become an issue for you based on the stage of Parkinson's that you're currently in but, rest assured, at some point it will become an issue for pretty much anyone with this disease. Coming right off the heels about the topic of drinking enough water, I wish I could say with certainty that doing so would resolve the issue every time, but unfortunately, it isn't quite that simple.

Constipation hits Parkinson patients particularly hard because of the damage the disease inflicts upon the autonomic nervous system, which is responsible for regulating the normal muscle activity associated with bowel movements. As time progresses and this system becomes ravaged by the disease, the muscles begin to slow down and digestion and bowel movements suffer. Hurting matters even more is having a low fluid intake, poor dietary choices, a sedentary lifestyle and even taking certain medications.

If you read the medical jargon you'll see recommendations for the usual remedies for constipation such as drinking plenty of water, prune juice, rigorous exercise and eating plenty of fiber. But sometimes, even that isn't enough because you aren't just dealing with your classic constipation symptoms here. These symptoms are much more intense because of Parkinson's.

Through trial and error, I've found something that works well for me so I'm passing it on to you. It's Citrucel, the orange-colored powder similar to Metamucil. The reason I chose it over the other brands is because it's the only variety that is gluten-free, which is a necessity for me because of my sensitivity to gluten. As long as I take this once in the morning and once in the evening, my system pretty much stays regular. Miss a dosage and I pay for it.

Your choices of food have a lot to do with whether or not you stay regular, too. Eating foods which are high in fat, contain dairy and sugar, foods that are fried and large amounts of protein might not affect the average non-Parkinson person, but for someone with the disease, it's a definite drawback. Also, certain foods such as bananas can encourage constipation. Of course, if you have a sensitivity to certain foods and especially gluten, you can naturally expect to have plenty of trouble if you partake of these things.

While some people may choose to turn to laxatives for relief, in many cases this isn't a viable option long-term, depending on the product. Some laxatives are only meant to relieve constipation for a short period of time and should not be adopted as a way of life. There are several reasons why they can be harmful if they are used for an extended period of time:

- they can cause an electrolyte imbalance, which can morph into abnormal heart rhythms
- they can interfere with the absorption of your medication
- they can disrupt the absorption of vitamins and nutrients from the foods that you eat
- they can actually train your colon to become less effective on it's own
- they can make you feel dizzy, lightheaded and confused

If you want to stick with a age-old remedy you can also try prune juice to alleviate your constipation. I've had good success with it, as well, but find it a little hard to get past the bitter taste. My wife's grandmother (she's 94) takes it every day, but adds a little sugar to it for taste. I've heard of some who make a little concoction out of 1 cup prune juice, 1 cup applesauce and 1 cup bran. Others have tried fiber gummy bears, which will be appealing for those with a sweet tooth.

Stress

We're all under a great deal of stress in our lives with things getting more stressful all the time. As if living day-to-day and cramming as much into as little time as possible wasn't stressful enough, those with Parkinson's disease see that stress level rise even higher because nothing is more stressful than having a daily struggle with a disease that you know you can't possibly cure.

But aside from Parkinson's, we have to take some of the responsibility for the fact that we bring a lot of our stress on ourselves. And it's not a hereditary pattern, either because we've managed to do this all on our own. Research has proven that today's adults are under more combined stress during a 30-day period than our grandparents were under *their entire lifetime combined.*

There are so many different kinds of stress attacking us on a regular basis that it's no wonder we feel pulled in so many directions:

1. Mental- working long hours, anxiety, worry, trying to do too much, being a perfectionist
2. Emotional- anger, resentment, hurt, sadness, fear, despair
3. Traumatic- being injured, sick, having surgery, extreme climate conditions
4. Physical- over-exerting yourself, performing physical labor, lack of sleep
5. Chemical- alcohol, tobacco, drugs, abusing prescription medications and other artificial stimulants
6. Environmental- pollutants, poor air quality, unfiltered drinking water, recirculated air
7. Nutritional- food allergies, poor nutrition
8. Personal- relationship issues, money worries
9. Professional- job stress, office politics, job security, commitments and deadlines, retirement worries

With this amount of stress coming at us from so many different directions it's no wonder we're constantly under stress. But while this is unhealthy for anyone, it's especially detrimental to someone with Parkinson's. It's just as important to focus attention on how Parkinson's affects you psychologically and emotionally as it does physically.

When you're under stress for a short period of time, your body responds accordingly by releasing cortisol (more on this later), which is the "fight or flight" hormone and adrenaline to help you combat the issue. But when you have Parkinson's disease, the resolution isn't that easy. You're already at a huge disadvantage because your disease has you under constant surveillance and a heightened degree of stress. Whenever your brain begins pumping out cortisol and adrenaline, it doesn't take much of it to seriously amplify your symptoms.

Stress, even minor stress, can exacerbate your symptoms, turning a simple hand tremor into a full-fledged arm movement. Even if you aren't experiencing tremors at the moment that the stress occurs, being exposed to stress can immediately cause tremors to begin and allow them to continue until the issue is resolved. If you're in public around others, the symptoms can be even worse because of the embarrassment associated with having tremors in front of others. This creates even more stress, which worsens tremors and so on and so on.

But while dealing with stress is bad enough it still isn't the worst part of stress. Science has proven that stress actually kills brain cells in the part of the brain called the hippocampus, which deals with memory, emotion and your autonomic nervous system. Not only that, but chronic stress does even more damage by prematurely aging your brain and making you much more susceptible to strokes. It can even lead to a condition known as adrenal fatigue, which I'll cover next.

Adrenal Fatigue

This condition has been known by many names throughout the years: neurasthenia, adrenal neurasthenia, sub-clinical hypoadrenia, non-Addison's hypoadrenia and, of course, the name you've probably heard it known by, adrenal fatigue. Although it is a very real and very complex condition, ironically, a vast majority of conventional medicine does not recognize it as an actual condition. So if you're looking for answers from your primary care doctor, good luck, because they probably either don't know much about it, aren't willing to listen to your symptoms with an open mind, or both.

When someone sees a conventional doctor complaining of the symptoms associated with adrenal fatigue, a conventional doctor will do what they do best which is to prescribe medication. Again, that's because they listen to your primary complaint (persistent fatigue) and they think that the answer lies in a prescription when, in fact, it has nothing to do the situation because you aren't suffering from a medication deficiency.

So what exactly is adrenal fatigue? Basically, it means that your adrenal glands (the small glands located directly above your kidneys) are tapped out. Your adrenal glands are responsible for supplying you with some very important hormones that your body requires in order for you to live. Two of these hormones are adrenaline and cortisol which, as we just covered, is the stress hormone.

The adrenals are responsible for monitoring hormones responsible for everything from managing your immune system and muscle tone to how your body regulates and stores energy all the way to regulating your heart rate, so as you can see they're pretty important. In other words, they maintain the proper balance of your internal environment (your body) in response to the external conditions.

When you develop adrenal fatigue, it means exactly as the name implies: that you have overpowered your adrenal glands with so much stress that they are no longer able to keep up with providing a reliable and sufficient supply of cortisol for your body's needs. It doesn't mean that they've completely shut down (or else you would be dead) but it does mean that they are only running at a fraction of their total efficiency.

Before I go any further, let's go back a step and see how stress plays in this scenario. When you're under stress, your body goes through a myriad of changes. The source of the stress can be physical (trauma to the body), emotional (a situation where you feel mentally torn) or psychological (death of a loved one). When your body experiences any stressful situation, it responds by increasing the heart rate and flooding your body with adrenaline and cortisol to combat the situation. Expose your body to a typical level of stress and your adrenals respond as they should by supplying you with the right amount of hormones. But if you expose them to either a single elevated level of stress or, more commonly, an extended period of stress, the glands are not able to keep up and they crash and burn.

Adrenal fatigue is sometimes hard to diagnose simply because it's hard to pinpoint a precise cause for what you're feeling. People with adrenal fatigue can sleep for eight hours and still wake up feeling exhausted. This is especially confusing for a Parkinson patient since we already feel that way on a regular basis.

Individuals with adrenal fatigue describe what they're experiencing by using phrases like "lack of interest" and that they "don't feel like themselves", although they're not exactly sure why. They find it necessary to use some sort of artificial stimulant(s) to keep them going just long enough to get them through the day. But, miraculously, in the evening around dinnertime, they suddenly feel a surge of energy, as if all of those stimulants that they tried during the day were stockpiled and finally decided to kick in all at once.

You're probably wondering how you can go from feeling like a slug to suddenly feeling like you have plenty of energy- and at the end of the day, no less. Logic would dictate that it should be the other way around with plenty of energy in the morning, seeing it gradually decline throughout the day and finally collapsing into sleep at bedtime. But that's how adrenal fatigue works. It means that your body's "clock" is off because your adrenal glands are mixed up.

When you first wake up, your glands are depleted and remain that way until right after lunch when you experience a slight rejuvenation from eating. But this is short-lived and by mid-afternoon, your cortisol naturally drops, which is called a diurnal drop, and you're back to downing caffeine to try to keep your eyelids propped open. By early evening, your adrenals have the ability to once again recover enough to give you another temporary boost, but even this spike tends to go away if you've experienced adrenal fatigue for some time.

If you listed them out, you could find upwards to 70 different symptoms that can be associated with adrenal fatigue, but since most of these only occur in a few people, I'm only going to touch on the ones that you're likely to see the most often.

Besides difficulty waking up, morning fatigue and higher energy levels in the evening, other symptoms commonly associated with adrenal fatigue include a craving for salty or sugary foods (I'll talk about why this happens in the next paragraph), dark circles under the eyes, difficulty handling stress, low blood pressure, low libido, a weakened immune system, trouble concentrating, low blood sugar and poor circulation.

Why is one of the symptoms an attraction to salty or sugary foods? Because one of the hormones produced in the adrenal is called aldosterone, a mineralocorticoid which works in synch with your kidneys to help them regulate proper fluid retention and mineral excretion. When you have adrenal fatigue, your cortisol levels aren't the only thing that drops- so does your level of aldosterone.

With your adrenals are shot, your body begins to excrete more and more minerals out in your urine. This is important because they just so happen to be minerals that are important to the body and shouldn't be leaving in the first place. The result is your body begins to have a difficult time balancing key minerals, such as sodium, magnesium, potassium and even glucose, leaving you with a craving for someone salty, sweet or, in many cases, both.

I need to make it clear that just because you might have all or even most of these symptoms doesn't automatically mean that you have adrenal fatigue so I don't want you to think that I'm trying to diagnose anyone. I'm only relaying what I've learned from mine and my wife's own personal experiences. If you suspect that you might be a victim of adrenal fatigue then that's where testing comes in.

Unfortunately, as is the case with Parkinson's disease there are no definitive tests which will clearly state without a doubt that "yes" you have adrenal fatigue or "no", you do not. However, if you can find the right kind of doctor, there are some tests that will contribute a great deal of information that can be used to help determine if adrenal fatigue is a possibility and to point them in the right direction of treatment. The most common of these tests is a saliva test, but others that can also be used include an AM cortisol test or an ACTH stimulation test. Besides these results, your doctor will also have to rely on a clinical evaluation and your medical history starting with your first sign of symptoms.

Most conventional doctors will dismiss the accuracy of these tests, citing that they are inconclusive to determining whether your adrenals are properly functioning. But remember, these are the same professionals who don't even recognize adrenal fatigue as an actual condition. They also don't believe in alternative methods of treatments, either, so you'll have to look elsewhere if you want to treat this naturally. And if you asked any of them about taking specific supplements in lieu of prescription medications, you'd get the "deer caught in the headlights" look because they're clueless about those, too.

I was fortunate in that my wife found a functional medicine doctor (who just so happens to also be a practicing chiropractor) who did saliva testing. When my results came back there was no question in her mind what was going on because they screamed adrenal fatigue. After being placed on the proper protocol, I saw an amazing improvement in my symptoms within just a short period of time. Besides cleaning up my eating habits, she also recommended I read up on adrenal fatigue which is where we found something else called an adrenal cocktail.

Adrenal cocktail

It might have a funny-sounding name, but don't let the name fool you because I'm here to tell you the results are serious.

My wife first introduced me to this drink shortly after I was first diagnosed because I was having such a hard time with being fatigued all the time. Even if you took the fact that I wasn't sleeping well out of the equation, I still didn't have anywhere near what could be considered a reasonable amount of energy. It didn't seem to matter how long I spent in the bed, I still never felt rested. It was as if my sleep wasn't being credited to my energy level the following day. I didn't want to go on yet another prescription, but I also didn't know what else to do. Thank goodness my wife intervened and found a functional medicine doctor who started us down the right path to recovery.

The adrenal cocktail consists of only three ingredients:

- 1/2 cup orange juice
- 1/4 teaspoon Himalayan salt
- 1/4 teaspoon Cream of Tartar

Mix well and drink. It might not sound like a viable combination of ingredients, but trust me, you don't want to knock it until you've tried it. I'll be the first one to admit that I was a little skeptical about the mixture, but after I tried it for the first time I was pleasantly surprised. Ideally, it's best if you do it twice a day (morning and late afternoon) around an hour before or after a meal.

Why these specific ingredients? Can Himalayan salt be substituted with regular sea salt? No. The specific reason behind why it has to be Himalayan salt is because this particular salt contains many of the minerals that we've been depleted of so it gives you an immediate boost of many of the things we're already deficient in. Himalayan salt is considered by many to be the purest form of salt on the planet and contains all of the 84 elements that you'll find in the human body.

The Cream of Tartar is actually potassium bitartrate, which works to help balance out your body's pH levels. Your body's pH levels refer to it's "potential Hydrogen" balance and is rated on a scale from 0 to 14, with 7 being the middle. Since our blood has a very narrow window for what it considers to be an acceptable pH level (7.35-7.45), anything outside of that tiny window means that you're sick. If pH levels become too far off (say, below 6.8 or above 7.8) then your body's cells stop working altogether.

Orange juice is used because not only is it packed with tons of vitamin C, but it also contains potassium, folate, thiamin and flavonoids, all very important for good health. It also has a powerful antioxidant called hesperidia (don't worry about experiencing a strange mixture of flavors because you really only taste the orange juice). While the adrenal cocktail primarily works on boosting your energy level, this combination of ingredients also reduces stress and can even help fight depression and anxiety.

Oxidative Stress

While stress as a whole is not good for us one of the worst examples of it is called oxidative stress. In the simplest of terms, this type of stress occurs when the body doesn't have enough antioxidants available to offer sufficient protection. Protection from what, you might ask? From free radicals.

Free radicals are nasty little creatures that have a Jekyll and Hyde complex. Ironically, they're actually useful in some instances while being completely destructive at other times. When our bodies process the oxygen that we breathe, our cells utilize it and produce energy from it, a process called oxidation. During oxidation, free radicals are created to conduct repairs. It's when the number of free radicals produced becomes too great that they begin to overwhelm our bodies and change from being an asset to suddenly becoming a liability.

When free radicals are unwarranted, these unstable molecules' sole purpose is to damage your cells. If a sufficient amount of antioxidants are available, then free radicals are kept at bay. Antioxidants achieve this by robbing free radicals of the electron that is responsible for giving them their destructive powers. But if antioxidant levels drop because of poor diet choices, then the body is an easy target for free radicals to seek out and destroy anything they come into contact with.

When free radicals are unopposed, cell membranes begin to age prematurely, which means *you* age prematurely. This can be seen as wrinkles, gray hair, poor eyesight, muscle and joint pain, fatigue, memory loss and arthritis. We typically accept these factors as a sign that we're getting older, but in reality it isn't just a natural occurrence and there is a perfectly logical reason behind why they're happening.

Another thing that happens as a result of out-of-control free radicals is that important enzymes in our bodies fall victim. In short, your entire DNA is negatively impacted. These free radicals seek out cells and either destroy them or mutate them into abnormal ones. By abnormal, we mean turning them into such things as heart disease, Alzheimer's disease and cancers. So you can see why keeping oxidative stress under control as much as possible is well worth the effort.

You're probably asking yourself what all this has to do with Parkinson's. Well, it has everything to do with it. As I mentioned, oxidative stress damages your cells, causing them to prematurely age. This increases a person's risk of developing Parkinson's. But just because you already have Parkinson's doesn't mean you're out of the woods.

Free radicals, the by-product of oxidative stress, age the brain. And in the case of a Parkinson's patient, that aging takes place at an accelerated rate because the neurons are now more sensitive to oxidative damage. It doesn't help matters that as we age, our neurons are automatically exposed to higher levels of oxidative stress, making the need to eliminate free radicals more important than ever and to begin doing so as early on as possible.

What puts you at the highest risk of developing oxidative stress? Some common factors include, but are not limited to:

- alcohol
- dehydration
- excessive sugar intake
- food preservatives
- infections (fungal, viral or bacterial)
- artificial food coloring and preservatives
- pollution
- being exposed to chlorinated water (either drinking, bathing or swimming)
- ingesting toxic chemicals
- pesticides/herbicides
- cleaning supplies
- cigarette smoke
- being exposed to radiation
- consuming too much animal protein
- hydrogenated oils
- heating oils to high temperatures (heating past the smoke point means the oil starts producing toxic fumes and starts to

decompose, producing free radicals)

Now that you know what causes free radicals, it's even more important to know how to fight them. Of course, the most practical way to avoid free radicals altogether is to avoid coming into contact with any of the irritants or circumstances listed above. But if you're already past that point (which all of us usually are, to an extent), and the damage has been done, then the next best course of action is to try to undo as much of the damage as you possibly can. Here are some suggestions:

1. Clean up your life. Stay away from as many chemicals, additives, preservatives, artificial colors and flavors, toxins and cleaning products as you can. Buy organic products whenever you can- especially when it's personal products.

2. Eliminate artificial stimulants. Alcohol needs to go and cigarettes contain over 4,000 chemicals- including more than 400 toxins and 42 known cancer-causing carcinogens.

3. Stay healthy. When you're sick, your immune system is desperately fighting off free radicals.

4. Avoid sugar. If you aren't going to completely eradicate it from your diet, at least cut back on it as much as possible. The more sugar you ingest, the more oxidative stress you open your body up to.

Even if you commit to doing everything that is listed above, it's completely unreasonable to expect anyone to totally eradicate stress and toxins from their life. So you have to take things one step further to minimize your exposure to free radicals by incorporating antioxidants into your diet.

Eat antioxidant-rich foods, such as:

- tomatoes
- spinach
- cruciferous vegetables: kale, cabbage, collards and broccoli
- asparagus

- onions
- garlic
- berries
- kale
- beets
- nuts and seeds
- avocados
- green tea

Take antioxidant supplements:

vitamin C
vitamin D
vitamin E
vitamin B12
zinc
selenium
magnesium
methylfolate

Chapter 11

The Massive Importance of Sleep (and Why It's Such An Issue For Those Of Us With Parkinson's Disease)

Some people are hesitant to devote one-third of their existence to sleep, citing that life is too short and believing that it's a waste of time to spend that much time in the sack. In the case of Parkinson's, there is typically a big difference between how much sleep we need and how much we actually end up getting. While some Parkinson patients are naturally wired to be able to function on less sleep than others, most of us require a minimum of eight hours and sometimes even more in order to feel well-rested.

Some individuals can appear to function just fine on as little as five or so hours of sleep while others meander around like zombies unless they get a full ten hour's worth. This doesn't mean that the five-hour people are tougher or have a stronger will because, sooner or later, that lack of sleep is going to catch up to them in a big way and when it does, it's going to be disastrous. That's leads me to the next thing I wish I had known when I was first diagnosed:

Insight #9: How Difficult It Is To Get Good Sleep.

If you looked at the list of things that can prevent you from getting a good night's sleep, you'd see that there are over 70 different sleep disorders that can interrupt your shuteye- and that's without even taking Parkinson's into consideration. That one factor alone is plenty to be concerned about and dwarfs pretty much anything else you could imagine before you even begin to worry about the other 70 some odd situations that can cause a sleepless night. No one knows how difficult it is to get good sleep more than someone with Parkinson's (a close second would be the person who has to sleep in the bed with someone who has Parkinson's).

There is a massive difference between getting sleep and getting good, deep, quality sleep (which is what your body so desperately needs). Parkinson patients have it especially hard because there are so many symptoms that can interfere with their sleep patterns. Things like rigid movements and stiffness can make it difficult to find a comfortable position, nighttime urination disrupts sleep and even something as simple as changing positions can set off tremors that can awaken you. Your muscles may even involuntarily spasm, jolting you awake.

Nightmares are a very real and very intrusive problem because due to the fact that they are often brought on by the medications you take, there is very little you can do to escape them. It is rare that once nightmares become a routine that they will ever decrease in frequency and intensity on their own. If it comes to the point that they interrupt your sleep too much, your best bet is to talk to your doctor. They may end up switching your medication or prescribing something that will hopefully help you overpower the action-packed and seemingly very real thoughts that your brain is putting you through at night.

Some individuals with Parkinson's have an unhealthy approach to sleep. They feel as if they can burn the candle at both ends during the week and rack up surplus sleep on the weekends. But no matter how hard you try you can't stockpile sleep. Once you reach a sleep deficit, called "sleep debt", your body is forced to deal with that deficit. It's also believed that your need for sleep decreases as you get older. This is also not true. If anything, you might need even more.

As sleep problems go, they tend to be one of the earliest warning signs that something is amiss. Early on, we just aren't familiar enough with Parkinson's disease to know to put the two together. You could literally suffer for years with sleep issues before other symptoms begin to appear. All my life I had slept like a baby, but once I was diagnosed, I could go back in time and remember when my sleep started being affected which fell right in line with the other issues I was having.

When we sleep, our brains are busy cycling between REM (rapid eye movement) sleep and non-REM sleep. As per the name, REM sleep means your eyes are darting around in different directions. When we first close our eyes and drift off, we are in a non-REM phase of sleep where we aren't dreaming. Then, we slip into a phase of REM for a short period of time before we slip back into the non-REM phase. This back-and-forth pattern can repeat itself several times before we are in what would be considered a "deep sleep".

There are three phases of non-REM sleep:

- Stage 1: Even though your eyes are closed you can still be awakened easily without feeling any effects because you haven't begun to drift off.
- Stage 2: You've entered into a "light sleep" as your body prepares for you to go into a deeper sleep. If you wake up from this you'll still be able to grasp reality fairly quickly.
- Stage 3: The stage of "deep sleep". When you are awakened during this phase, you feel temporarily disoriented and groggy for a few minutes until you can once again get your bearings.

We have to be asleep for an average of 90 minutes before our bodies fall into the first episode of REM sleep. This only lasts for around 10 minutes before we change into a short period of non-REM, go back to REM and so on. But each episode of REM sleep is longer than the previous one, with the longest one lasting roughly an hour.

Why am I going to all the trouble of explaining this? Because not only do we dream during REM sleep but it is also during this time when we experience a phenomenon known as REM behavior disorder, or RBD. Once you hear it described, no doubt you'll recognize it and then you'll feel relieved to finally be able to put an actual name to what you've been going through.

Parkinson patients should recognize RBD right off the bat because if you're having difficulty staying asleep, chances are you might have this condition, courtesy of Parkinson's. When you have RBD, you tend to act out your dreams which can involve punching, kicking, talking in your sleep, yelling, screaming and even getting up out of the bed without waking. It can hit very quickly and scientists haven't been able to distinguish any rhyme or reason as to why some nights you can be more active in your sleep than others.

During REM sleep, our brain acts in a similar fashion to the way it does when we're awake. Someone who does not have Parkinson's but has RBD experiences muscle paralysis, so they can have vivid dreams and remain perfectly still. But a Parkinson patient isn't as fortunate, which is why we tend to move about so aggressively when we're supposed to be lying still and resting.

There have been studies which show 3 out of 4 people who suffer from RBD went on to develop Parkinson's. This isn't to say that if you have REM sleep issues you'll likely develop Parkinson's, but it does show that most Parkinson patients can recall a time in the past before being diagnosed when they saw a noticeable decrease in the quality of their sleep. Also, Parkinson patients are three times as likely to have some sort of motor restlessness of the legs than non-Parkinson individuals.

Parkinson's patients also have the unfortunate side effect of disrupted circadian rhythms. Since dopamine is directly connected to our circadian rhythms, and Parkinson's is all about a depletion of that dopamine, it stands to reason that having dopamine inefficiencies would cause disruptions in our sleep. When a Parkinson patient sleeps well, it's because there's been an improvement in dopaminergic functioning, or an increase in the amount of dopamine stored in the nigrostriatal terminals located in the brain.

For most Parkinson patients, myself included, the span of time from when you turn out the lights until you are able to fall asleep, known as sleep onset latency, isn't usually the problem. It is the sleep inefficiency or sleep fragmentation that results in the individual waking up over and over again during the night.

Besides experiencing and acting out vivid dreams, Parkinson patients routinely experience periodic leg movement disorder, or PLMD, which is where the patient tends to kick their partner in their sleep. This is also due to the acting out of dreams that the patient deems to be very realistic. Another common, and less aggressive disorder is leg restlessness where the patient randomly thrashes their legs about without any specific pattern, as if their legs are uncontrollably shaking or moving independently of the body. This is not to be confused with restless legs syndrome, or RLS, where the individual moves in an attempt to stop an uncomfortable sensation they are dreaming about.

Because of the difficulties with trying to get successive nights of good, quality sleep, Parkinson patients are much more likely to develop daytime fatigue, on top of the fatigue already generated by the disease. Being robbed of quality sleep- even occasionally- can cause Parkinson tremors to be worse. Adding to the mix are the side effects of medications that interrupt normal sleep patterns. When you add all of that together, we really have a lot of things working against our sleep.

As a Parkinson patient, sleep apnea may also be a major concern since 40 percent of patients experience it. Besides the stereotypical symptom of loud snoring, those who suffer from this condition will also suffer with restless sleep and have pauses in their breathing while sleeping. As you can imagine, this will also cause them to experience daytime fatigue and difficulty concentrating. Given the seriousness of this condition if you or your spouse suspects that you might have sleep apnea you should inform your doctor immediately.

The most common form of sleep apnea is called obstructive sleep apnea (OSA). Like those without Parkinson's who suffer with this sleeping disorder, OSA occurs when the soft walls of the throat collapse and obstruct the airway. The major difference is that unlike someone in the general population with OSA, a Parkinson's patient doesn't have to be overweight.

But the worst residual effect from not obtaining sound sleep is an increase in symptoms the following day. Fatigue exacerbates Parkinson symptoms, making it appear as if your medication's "on" and "off" times have been manipulated. This can make even the simplest of tasks much more difficult than they need to be.

How Much Sleep Do *You* Need?

Although we should all strive to get a minimum of 8 hours every night it isn't always that easy. In fact, with Parkinson's disease it's nearly impossible to determine so this answer varies from person to person. In order to ensure that you're getting enough sleep, you could try to assess how you feel during the day and if you notice feeling overly tired or sluggish, but this isn't really a fair way to gauge things since you could be supplementing you energy needs with some form of artificial stimulant. This false prop might have you thinking that you feel fine when your body is actually lacking in much-needed rest. If you want the most accurate measurement you have to ask yourself a few questions to determine if you're on target for the right quantity of sleep:

1. Do you require artificial stimulants at the beginning or the middle of the day just to make it through?
2. Do you feel a noticeable slump in your energy right after lunch?
3. Are you having weight issues or trouble losing weight?
4. Is it hard to stay awake when you're performing mundane tasks such as driving?
5. Do you get headaches when you haven't ever had a history of them before?
6. Are you easily agitated, have less patience and feel as if you're "on edge"?

It isn't feasible to try to put a blanket statement on all Parkinson patients and tell them exactly how much sleep they need because there is no set amount. But given the challenges that Parkinson patients have with sleep, it would be wise to learn as much about it as you can about ways to resolve it so you'll be better equipped to deal with the issue.

There are countless natural products on the market that people respond well to, many of which I'll cover later on in this chapter. You might have to go through a few before you come across one that helps and, even then, it might not completely alleviate the problem, but if it offers you some sort of relief then it's worth it. Your best bet is to stay away from prescriptions, if at all possible, so you don't risk taking something that might interfere with your Parkinson meds.

How Cortisol Plays A Major Role In Sleep

I briefly touched on cortisol in Chapter 10, but because of its relevance to getting good sleep I thought it required some further discussion.

As you know there are several common reasons why someone with Parkinson's can't get a good night's sleep. Topping this list are side effects from medications and, of course, stress. But when talking about stress, you can't be so simplistic about labeling it as a reason for not sleeping since there's much more to finding a remedy than just saying that you're going to try to reduce stress in your life. It involves much more than that since people with Parkinson's react differently to stress than those who don't have the disease.

When someone is under stress, their hypothalamic pituitary adrenal system, or the adrenal glands, for short, release the stress hormone cortisol. For your typical person, the cortisol goes to work to help the body fight through the stress. This release of cortisol is expected and well-received when it is released in moderation and everything functions as it should. It's when this release becomes a prolonged habit or occurs much too frequently that bad things start to happen.

Having that much excess cortisol begins to damage cells everywhere- up to and including those all-important neurons in the brain that are responsible for producing dopamine. This is where the damage stress causes differs for Parkinson's patients. When *we* are placed under stress and cortisol is released, things get even worse for us because our dopamine supplies are already greatly depleted, therefore, the amount of damage inflicted hits us harder- and that's just under normal stressful conditions. Imagine how much greater damage we're subjecting ourselves to from repeated or prolonged periods of stress.

How Depression Influences Cortisol

It is a well-documented fact that depression often accompanies Parkinson's. Patients are in a constant fight to prevent it from overpowering their lives all while it is desperately trying to find one of the many ways to force itself in so it can wreak havoc.

With so much to worry about it's no wonder Parkinson patients can succumb to depression so often. We can become depressed because of the limitations that have been forced upon us, the financial obligations that come with it, a less-than-desirable prognosis, the constant regimen of medications that we must endure, other medical complications that we've experienced as a result of Parkinson's or merely the fact that we even have Parkinson's. All of that depression compounds and works together to takes its toll on our health.

We already know that the release of cortisol caused by stress damages the hypothalamus portion of the brain and we know that cortisol release can, and often does, lead to depression. But what most people don't see is that when you put either excess cortisol or depression into a scenario of someone with Parkinson's disease, your circadian rhythms are disrupted and you have fractured sleep patterns.

So imagine what happens when cortisol and depression act together. Now you have a Parkinson's patient who already has trouble sleeping, has increased cortisol levels due to stress (which can easily be from not sleeping) and, on top of that, is depressed. How on earth could anyone be expected to sleep while trying to fight off *that* kind of an attack?

Having a combination of depression and elevated cortisol are not a fluke. If you took a close look at all of the individuals who are depressed, both with and without Parkinson's disease, you'd find an elevated amount of cortisol in roughly half of them. It's relatively easy for the body to dispense excess cortisol in these situations because the brain thinks it's doing something good when, in actuality, it isn't- even though it's running purely out of instinct.

Depression does an excellent job of masking what the true cortisol levels are in your body, allowing for more and more of the hormone to be pumped into your system despite the fact that you've already achieved sufficient levels with which to handle the "crisis".

Research shows that people who suffer from depression do not conform to the typical guidelines that the body uses to determine when cortisol should be released. Although depressed individuals do have specific times of the day that their brain releases cortisol, it isn't during optimal times. Someone without depression will see their cortisol levels at their highest around 8 AM and 4 PM with the lowest level recorded in the middle of the night while they're sleeping. But depressed individuals can see levels spiking at the most inopportune times- especially during the middle of the night when they're trying to rest.

Why is there such a mix-up of communication in these instances? It can all be blamed on the hypothalamus, the portion of your brain that gets the ball rolling in releasing cortisol.

The hypothalamus is not only responsible for regulating the pituitary glands, but it also uses neurotransmitters to work in synch with your endocrine system to regulate many of our body's activities, including sleep. These neurotransmitters include norepinephrine, serotonin and, you guessed it, dopamine.

The process of releasing cortisol is a simple one. It all starts in the hypothalamus where corticotropin-releasing hormone (CRH), also known as corticotropin-releasing factor (CRF), is released in order to stimulate the adrenal gland into releasing it's own contribution to the cause, the adrenocorticotrophic hormone, or ACTH. Once ACTH is put into action, this signals the adrenal glands to begin releasing cortisol out into the blood to begin the fight.

Under normal conditions, the timing is impeccable and everything works as it was designed as the hypothalamus keeps a close eye on cortisol levels, increasing and decreasing its release as needed. When cortisol levels increase, the hypothalamus tells the pituitary gland to lower its production of CRF. Likewise, when cortisol drops, CRF production increases. But when a person experiences depression, everything changes. When this happens, that instinctive signaling is interrupted and the hypothalamus is no longer accurately measuring levels of cortisol.

This causes the hypothalamus to erroneously tell the pituitary gland to keep supplying cortisol, even though levels are already much too high. In short, this is how depression can be responsible for elevating cortisol levels, which then impede sleep. And since excess cortisol damages the hypothalamus, the very same area that is necessary in order to properly monitor cortisol, these signals continue to be disrupted, placing your brain on a runaway train towards disaster.

Ways To Improve Your Sleep

We're all aware of how prescription sleep medications usually come with side effects. Sometimes the side effects are worse than experiencing a lack of sleep because they tend to cross over into the following day, leaving us groggy, sluggish and fighting to get a firm hold on our day. Wouldn't it be better to deal with your sleep issues in a more natural way that is less likely to make matters worse for you? If you'd prefer to find a healthier option for treating your sleep problems then here are a few suggestions that actually work for many:

Acupuncture. Before you dismiss it, you have to consider the validity of this practice since it's been around for literally thousands of years. It uses tiny needles (no, they don't hurt going in) to tap into energy flows inside the body called "meridians". When these flows of energy become blocked by different form of stress (stress from food, disease, depression, inflammation, etc.), your body responds with symptoms. The specific meridians opened for Parkinson's patients help to release both serotonin and tryptophan. It might take more than one session, but it's very effective.

Get the right pillow. Chiropractors everywhere will tell you that if your head, neck and spine aren't lined up correctly while you're lying down then you're putting unnecessary strain on your neck and shoulder muscles which causes them to tense and cramp (even if you might not be aware of it). This constant, albeit mild tension, can subconsciously prevent you from properly relaxing enough to fall into a deep, restful sleep.

Here's the test to see if you're aligned properly: have someone stand next to your bed while you lie down on your side and then on your back to see if your spine is in alignment. If it isn't, then you're placing unnecessary stress on your neck and shoulder muscles, meaning that it's time to switch out your pillow.

Aromatherapy. Although its uses are broad, it makes for an excellent sleep aid. This isn't a bunch of woo-woo nonsense. Aromatherapy really works and there are countless studies to prove it. By far, the best scent to use is lavender with jasmine, sandalwood and chamomile rounding out the list. You can either use a diffuser or place a sachet of the preferred scent next to your pillow.

L-Theanine, or Theanine. A main component of green tea, it works by increasing alpha wave activity, which, in turn, promotes calmness. It's ability to cross over between the brain/blood barrier makes it an excellent choice for reducing stress and anxiety since this barrier is often the barricade that prevents many supplements, and even some prescription anxiety medications, from gaining access to the brain where they can go to work and perform their intended purpose. Simply chew two tablets 30 minutes before bedtime and drift off to sleep once you feel the calmness overtaking you.

Don't exercise right before bed. When you exercise, your body releases adrenaline- the *last* thing you want hanging around right before bedtime.

Wild lettuce. No, this isn't the name of a vegetarian rock band: it's a supplement that helps with headaches, joint and muscle pain, anxiety and helping you relax, so there are many ways it can be beneficial to you. It's also been shown to help with restless leg syndrome.

Tart cherry juice. Cherry juice is full of tryptophan, the amino acid that first converts to serotonin and then converts over to melatonin. It's best known as the infamous ingredient in turkey that always makes you sleepy after a Thanksgiving meal. But it has to be the "tart" variety since regular cherry juice contains way too much sugar.

Hyland's Calm Tablets. They're all-natural, non habit-forming and, best of all, inexpensive. You can either take a couple of them 30-60 minutes before bedtime to improve sleep or you can use them during the day if you're experiencing an overly-stressful time.

Keep your bedroom just a bedroom. This room should be your sanctuary, not a place for the treadmill, a desk or anything else that is going to take away from the atmosphere of relaxation. You're supposed to come in there for refuge so if you have to, clean it out and make it peaceful-looking.

Valerian root. Another great sleep aid that imposes a soothing effect by increasing the amount of GABA (gamma aminobutyric acid), which helps to promote calmness by regulating nerve cells. But here's a fair warning: you'll want it in a capsule form because of the unpleasant smell.

St. John's Wort. Typically recommended for depression, it works by increasing serotonin levels, which, in turn, means more melatonin allowing you to sleep better.

"White" noise machines. Sometimes when we're trying to sleep, we get distracted by the sounds around us (pets, passing traffic, the weather, etc). These machines create artificial or "white" noise to mask the noises around you so you can concentrate on staying asleep. They come with different volume settings and different noises (ocean waves, rustling brook, nighttime sounds in the country and even the low murmur of a crowded restaurant, just to name a few). I've used them for years and I wouldn't trade mine for gold. I'm a very light sleeper and something as simple as our dog re-positioning herself on the carpeted floor wakes me.

Limit "screen" time. Watching electronics fires up your brain and keeps it excited for quite some time afterwards. You should limit computer time to at least an hour before you're ready for bed to give your brain time to calm back down.

OTC sleep aids. I'm not opposed to trying whatever works but if you find one that helps be prepared for the effects to lessen as time goes on and our bodies adjust to it.

Add in some nutmeg. No, you didn't read that wrong. The spice that you bake with can also help you sleep.

Nutmeg just so happens to contain the amino acid tryptophan, the same nap-inducing ingredient that you'll find in your Thanksgiving turkey. Add 1/8 of a teaspoon into a cup of warm milk before bed and let it kick in.

One Thing You Shouldn't Try

Melatonin. Melatonin is the serotonin-derived hormone, which helps modulate our sleep patterns. It's secreted by the pea-sized pineal gland located in the brain. Under normal conditions, this secretion automatically takes place as we approach bedtime, causing us to naturally become drowsy. But since there is so much inconsistency within the brains of Parkinson patients, that secretion doesn't take place as it should. As a result, we often have trouble falling asleep. The most obvious answer to this dilemma would be to simply supplement the melatonin ourselves to make up the difference. Unfortunately, that really isn't a good idea.

Melatonin has been used for countless years as an effective and natural way to help you get a good night's sleep. It's unfortunate that Parkinson patients can't benefit from this option. Why? Because even though it has been shown to occasionally offer some improvement in sleep, there are countless studies which show that melatonin produces unfavorable motor effects by conflicting with the pathways that supply dopamine. Taking too much can actually increase the risk of depression and toxicity. There is also ample evidence about how melatonin interacts with medications and can disrupt your circadian rhythms. It's generally not even recommended for long-term use by those who *don't* have Parkinson's, much less those of us who do.

If you are committed to giving melatonin a try, you'll want to go with the sublingual versions, which are placed under the tongue, allowing them to enter the bloodstream much quicker. Before I was instructed by my doctor not to use them, this is the version I used. I placed two 5mg tablets under my tongue about 30 minutes before I was ready for bed and within a few minutes, they were dissolved. I admit that by bedtime I felt drowsiness coming on. It just didn't do a good enough job for me. But the key to using melatonin is to not force yourself to stay up past this point. When you begin to feel the effects, you need to succumb and go to sleep. If you try to push through and fight it, before you know it, the effects will begin to wear off and you'll be wide awake and right back at square one.

Chapter 12

The Incredible Power of Magnesium

There are so many things that Parkinson's patients can do to improve the quality of their lives while trying to keep this dreadful disease at bay, at least as much as humanly possible. Some are things that we're willing to try while others are things that we casually dismiss- usually because we don't know enough about it to give it a fair chance. But if there is one thing that you should sit up and take notice of, it's magnesium. In fact, it's so important that I've devoted an entire chapter to it just to try to convince you of how incredibly important this one mineral really is. My hope is that by the end of this chapter, you'll see why I'm such a proponent of it.

Although the numbers range, statistics show that up to 80 percent (possibly even more) of us are magnesium deficient. Why is that number so high? There are several reasons. The first can be blamed on the Standard American Diet, which doesn't really allow magnesium consumption since it's based on white flour, dairy and meat- none of which contain magnesium. The second reason is the fact that most people don't know how important it is for us to have- particularly if you have Parkinson's.

If you're still questioning whether or not it's something worth looking into, let me approach it from a scientific viewpoint. There are no accidental minerals present in the body. Each mineral that our body contains has a reason for being there and, therefore, has its own distinct properties. Each also has it's own characteristic electrical charge, called a valance. In order to measure the valance, or the electrical charge of a mineral, you have to dissolve the mineral in fluid. When you take a look at every mineral found in our bodies, magnesium has the highest valance of all of them.

What does this mean? It means that magnesium isn't your typical run-of-the-mill nutrient. It's responsible for over *300* different enzymatic reactions in the body. Here are just a few of the most important things it does for you:

- synthesizes fatty acids and proteins
- enables enzymes to function properly
- breaks down glucose
- regulates the production of cholesterol
- metabolizes food
- relaxes muscles
- aids in digestion
- activates adenosine triphosphate (ATP) in the body, which produces energy
- is used as a foundation for RNA (protein)

Enzymes are the molecules that allow the body to perform all of the functions that it was designed to carry out. But enzymes aren't able to do this by themselves. They also need what are called enzyme co-factors. Co-factors act as a guide for the enzymes to carry out their duties with magnesium being the quintessential co-factor.

But magnesium does so much more that should be of specific interest to Parkinson's patients:

It helps your bones. Between 50 and 60 percent of the magnesium in your body is found in your bones. When magnesium levels are too low, it sets off a chain reaction starting with a drop in your parathyroid hormone, or PTH. Your PTH is essentially responsible for the amount of calcium found in bones and actually bonds to the very cells, which are responsible for creating bone in the first place. PTH also helps your kidneys and intestines retain more calcium. When the intestines and kidneys aren't retaining sufficient levels of calcium, guess where that much-needed calcium ends up? In the toilet- literally.

It helps lower inflammation. By suppressing a major inflammation trigger called interleukin 1, magnesium lowers your risk of developing a multitude of medical issues, all of which stem from inflammation (which was discussed in chapter 9). If you look at the complete list, there are over *3,500* conditions that can be directly tied to a magnesium deficiency.

It helps stabilize your DNA. Our body's genetic code, known as deoxyribonucleic acid, or DNA, requires magnesium as one of its chief building blocks. Even though a typical cell has a lifespan of approximately 7 years, they die off at a continuous rate, and, therefore, must be replaced.

It boosts energy. In order for our body to produce energy from the foods that we take in, there are many different chemical reactions that have to take place within the body. All of these reactions are not only necessary, but they have to be timed perfectly and in-synch with each other in order for this to work. Magnesium is a major contributor to ensuring that these reactions all take place exactly when they're supposed to.

It helps you sleep. When magnesium levels drop, so does melatonin. At the same time, magnesium helps control stress, which can also interfere with sleep.

It helps keep teeth healthy. When someone is deficient in magnesium, calcium and phosphorus levels also go out of balance. These imbalances collect in the saliva where they damage teeth.

It helps your heart (in several ways). First, it helps strengthen the most important muscle in the body, the heart (25 percent of the magnesium in your body is found in your muscles), while also strengthening blood vessels. The second way it benefits you heart is because it is a natural blood thinner.

It may help lower your cancer risk. Recent studies show that every 100mg increase in magnesium lowered the risk of colorectal cancer by more than 10 percent.

How Magnesium Boosts Your Nervous System

Next to a pumping heart, your central nervous system is the most important component in your entire body. Every function of the human body requires an electrical current in order to occur. Calcium is the principal conductor which allows all of these electrical currents to take place and since we already know that magnesium is responsible for maintaining proper calcium levels, you can see how magnesium has such a dramatic and positive impact on your nervous system.

Magnesium regulates calcium in your body using a simple system. Like an electrical current in your home, the electrical currents in your body also require both negative and positive charges. Magnesium and calcium are both positively charged while the majority of nerve tissues are negatively charged. Since our nerves are constantly trying to "discharge", or lose their power, they need the combination of magnesium and calcium to maintain a charge and allow current (nerve impulses) to occur.

Another way to look at your central nervous system is to compare it to a battery. A battery requires both a positive and a negative charge in order to provide power. Since negative energy is always present in a battery that means that a dead battery is the result of all of the positive energy being lost or depleted. In the case of the battery, being depleted means that it won't run anything. In the case of your central nervous system, being depleted means that your nerves start to misfire.

Here's how it works: located in all of our cell membranes are a special type of molecules called receptors. These membrane receptors are responsible for both sending and receiving chemical messages. When you look at the brain, the hub of the central nervous system, you'll find the most important membrane receptor of all, the N-methyl-d-aspartate, or NMDA receptor, as it is commonly called. This receptor is the part of the brain affected when you are put under anesthesia. It also happens to be the part of the brain, which can trigger depression when NMDA receptors are low. So, in other words, when your magnesium is low your NMDA receptors are low and you're much more prone to depression.

Magnesium has such an impact on nerves that it is often used as an anti-depressant, as well as a treatment for seizures, convulsions and recovering alcoholics. It's also given to pregnant women who suffer for pre-eclampsia (high blood pressure).

If you've been paying attention, you're probably wondering how magnesium can boost energy *and* simultaneously have a calming effect at the same time, right? After all, you'd think it would have to be one or the other, but not both. It does this by stamping out fatigue while allowing your natural energy to be utilized. You see, you don't always have to give up one for the other.

For example, science has shown us that hibernating animals have extremely high levels of magnesium in their systems- even after months of continuous sleeping. But if you woke up a hibernating bear, it would have the ability to immediately run you down with very little effort, despite the fact that it hasn't eaten in months. Logic dictates that the bear should be so weak that it wouldn't even have the energy to stand up, much less take off on a dead run. So, you see, you can be relaxed and *still* have the energy that you need.

So Why Are We So Deficient?

Besides making poor food choices, there are many things we do which bring down magnesium levels that we aren't even aware of:

- high salt intake: substitute cheap table salt for Celtic sea salt or Himalayan salt
- alcohol
- profuse sweating
- prolonged periods of stress
- consuming phosphoric acid (found in carbonated drinks)
- medications- specifically antibiotics
- coffee
- chronic diarrhea
- diuretics

But even if you avoided all of these issues, that's still no guarantee that your magnesium levels would remain optimal because you have two very important issues working against you. Not only does your body not retain magnesium easily, it also has a difficult time absorbing it, as well. That means being on constant alert and diligent about getting enough magnesium.

Generations ago, we didn't have to worry as much about supplementing magnesium because good old Mother earth took care of it for us by supplying us with magnesium-rich soil for growing crops. But you can no longer rely on getting a reasonable quantity of magnesium from our soil, as in the good old days, because erosion and contamination of our soil from pesticides and herbicides have depleted much of the natural magnesium that was once found there. Other things that contribute to a reduction in magnesium in the soil is acid rain and fertilizers containing potash, which is preferred by and, subsequently, absorbed by plants instead of the magnesium and calcium that they should be pulling from the ground.

We have other ways in which we unknowingly work to keep magnesium levels down:

1. Stress. The more your stress levels go up, the more your hydrochloric acid and stomach acids go down, preventing the absorption of magnesium. The same goes for antacid products, which are specifically designed to cut hydrochloric acid. The truth is antacid products do more harm than good because they not only kill off the bad acids in your gut, but they eliminate the good acids, too. This is a problem because your gut needs those good acids so it can break down your food.

If you need to take antacid products then there's something else going on that needs to be addressed. Cutting back on stomach acid isn't the answer. All you're doing is getting rid of the good along with the bad, which is going to turn your digestive system upside down because you have to have enough hydrochloric acid in your gut to break down your food. That's why I take Zypan with my meals when I'm having protein.

2. Having fluoride in our water supplies and toothpaste. Not only does fluoride bind to magnesium and makes it unavailable to be absorbed and used by the body, but the fluoride actually takes the place of magnesium in our bones and cartilage.

Approximately half of all fluoride that you ingest ends up in your bones while the remaining fluoride is excreted in our urine. Once it settles into our bones, it sets up home for quite a while. In fact, it takes about *2 decades* for your body to eliminate just *half* of the fluoride that has concentrated in your bones- and that's only if you haven't ingested any more fluoride within the last 20 years, which, I'm sure you'll agree, is next to impossible. That means that you're constantly adding more fluoride to bones that are already heavily saturated with it. That means that you're fighting a losing battle.

What does all that excess fluoride do to you? Well, for starters, it interferes with the body's natural ability to rebuild bone. It can also cause a calcification of your joints and the development of arthritis. But, as if that wasn't bad enough, probably the biggest issue you'll face is what it does to your kidneys.

As we age, our kidneys start to run less efficiently. Since we're relying on them to dispose of the unabsorbed half of the fluoride we're taking in, that puts an extra unnecessary strain on our kidneys, which are already having a hard enough time keeping up with the demands being placed on them. That leaves you in a bad predicament because not only are you absorbing a tremendous amount of fluoride into your bones, but the only way that your body has of eliminating some of it has been jeopardized.

3. Low potassium. Also known as hypokalemia, this causes the body to flush out more magnesium than it should.

4. Processed foods. Whenever you mill flour, you're, in essence, removing magnesium. Even vegetables containing magnesium aren't necessarily safe. Anytime you boil them, they lose magnesium.

5. Junk food. They use up too much magnesium. This especially goes for sugary foods.

6. Eating high trans and saturated fats. Both of these intensify the walls of cells, making it more difficult for magnesium to be absorbed into them.

7. Other medical conditions. Having leaky gut syndrome, irritable

bowel syndrome (IBS), an allergy to casein or gluten or parasites all deplete magnesium supplies.

Symptoms of Magnesium Deficiency

Even though there are quite a few classic symptoms that scream a deficiency in magnesium, they are often ignored because they also happen to be classic symptoms of other common medical conditions. To avoid any possibility of confusion, here are the standard symptoms of magnesium deficiency:

- fatigue
- insomnia
- headaches
- sugar cravings
- asthma
- foggy thinking
- anxiety/panic attacks
- hypertension
- irritability
- weakness
- depression
- bowel diseases
- nausea and vomiting
- muscle cramps
- heart palpitations

With the similarities between a magnesium deficiency and other common ailments being so close, it's important to let you doctor know as soon as you begin to experience any of these symptoms so they can take the necessary steps to pinpoint exactly what the cause is.

How To Increase Magnesium Levels

You probably think that solving the issue of being deficient in magnesium is easily remedied by just boosting your magnesium, right? Well, yes and no.

While it's a good effort to focus on boosting your magnesium, there's more to the problem than just that one mineral. The only way to properly boost your magnesium is to focus on other important nutrients that are tied directly to magnesium and work together with it as a team in order to achieve a more perfect balance in the body. There are three additional nutrients that you should consider if you want to achieve the best results. They are:

- calcium
- vitamin K2
- vitamin D

Why is it so important that these three nutrients be lumped together with magnesium? Because they are the most effective as a team.

Every one of us has heard about how we need sufficient calcium for strong bones and teeth since elementary school. But there is such a thing as having too much calcium, a condition known as hypercalcemia. If you're already experiencing issues with having too much calcium, you might be interested to know that having low magnesium just amplifies the problem even more. But there's much more at stake than just compromised bones because hypercalcemia can be a very serious condition. And since we tend to consume more calcium than we should, on top of the fact that we're probably already deficient in magnesium, the likelihood that we'll develop hypercalcemia goes up dramatically.

Vitamin K2 comes into the picture because it actually has the unique ability of being able to help control calcium. However, when vitamin K2 isn't readily available in ample quantities to police calcium, the excess calcium begins to make its way to places it shouldn't go, like your soft tissue, for example. That kind of buildup leads to muscle cramping, osteoarthritis, kidney stones, insomnia and constipation (how about that, Parkinson patients) and an increased risk for cancer of the prostate and breast. Calcium buildup can also cause an accumulation of plaque in your arteries and put unnecessary stress on your heart.

But hold on. You can also easily overdo it with too much calcium without even adding vitamin K2 into the equation. Trying to ramp up your calcium intake too much allows the excess calcium to become stored in your bones until the body tells it that it's needed. That might sound like good news, but it really isn't.

This is another prime example of "more is not better". The cells responsible for building new bone, called osteoblasts, are constantly trying to keep up with osteoclasts, which are responsible for breaking down a portion of old bones so they can be rebuilt. Calcium disrupts the work done by the builders, the osteoblasts, allowing the osteoclasts to accelerate their demolition of bones. The result? Your bones are broken down faster than they can be rebuilt.

The last of the three nutrients that are vital to supporting magnesium is vitamin D. Having adequate vitamin D levels is crucial for both magnesium absorption and retention. But since most individuals, both with and without Parkinson's, are already deficient in vitamin D, this isn't a reasonable line of support to rely on all by itself. Once again, if you only focus on ramping up your vitamin D and neglect the importance of calcium and vitamin K2, you're only hurting yourself and, in the long run you can even end up experiencing vitamin D toxicity.

If you want to get the majority of your magnesium from what you eat, here are the foods, in descending order from highest to lowest levels, that contain the most magnesium:

- pumpkin seeds
- spinach
- Swiss chard
- soybeans
- sesame seeds
- quinoa
- black beans
- cashews
- sunflower seeds
- navy beans
- pinto beans
- Lima beans

If you aren't a particular fan of these foods then your only other option to get your recommended amount of magnesium is to supplement it.

How much magnesium should you be getting?

- males- 350 mg/day
- females- 280mg/day (if you're pregnant or lactating, that number goes up to 350 mg/day)

Types of Magnesium To Try

As you can probably imagine, there are countless varieties of magnesium supplements being sold. Simply running to your nearest vitamin store and asking for a magnesium supplement isn't going to be sufficient because there are so many different types of magnesium available that it's rather easy to make a mistake and pick one that isn't going to do you as much good as you deserve. That's why it's important to understand what these varieties are and how they differ because each variety has it's own special properties that make it unique from the others. Below are the most common, and most helpful ones to be on the lookout for:

Magnesium glycinate. This type of magnesium is combined with the non-essential amino acid, glycine, hence the name. It's generally considered to be the safest option for anyone who has a long-term history of being magnesium-deficient simply because it is the least likely of all the varieties to upset your stomach (a very important factor that you'll find out about once you begin taking a magnesium supplement).

Magnesium citrate. By far, the most popular of the magnesium supplement family due to the fact that it's so readily absorbed into the bloodstream. It's also very inexpensive. I use a variety called "Natural Calm". It comes in powder form and you simply mix it with cold or warm water (cold water gives it a spritzer kind of taste, but warm water reminds me too much of Alka Seltzer).

You can use up to two teaspoonfuls of magnesium citrate at a time without worry that you're getting too much. But let me give you fair warning about an added bonus: the citric acid in this makes it a natural laxative (I already hear all of the constipated Parkinson's patients cheering), so if you jump out there and try two teaspoonfuls right off the bat, you'll might end up with loose stools- depending on how deficient your body is. The best way to start out is with one teaspoonful and, if you do okay, slowly ramp it up to two teaspoonfuls over the course of a week or two.

Magnesium taurate. This is the recommended choice for individuals who have a history of cardiovascular issues. Besides being absorbed easily into the bloodstream, it also doesn't have a laxative effect to it.

Magnesium malate. If you're suffering from fatigue, using this variety of magnesium will kill two birds with one stone by boosting both your energy and you magnesium levels. The secret is the malic acid, which is the fruit acid that naturally occurs in the body when carbs are converted over to energy. The collective enzymes of malic acid make it a perfect building block for creating adenosine triphosphate (ATP), which transports energy to your cells to feed your metabolism and for producing energy.

Magnesium chloride. Although it contains the last amount of elemental magnesium of all the varieties (somewhere around 12 perfect), it still has several things going for it. For one, it fires up your metabolism. Second, it's excellent for detoxing cells and tissue and third, it boosts kidney function.

Magnesium carbonate. This variety actually turns into magnesium chloride as soon as it hits your stomach acids. Since its antacid properties target your digestive system so well, this makes it a great aid for those who suffer from reflux and indigestion.

Magnesium sulfate (hydroxide). This is commonly known by its store shelf name: Epsom salt. You don't want to try to take this internally because it's very easy to overdose on it and then you'll just end up causing yourself more problems. However, taking a hot bath with Epsom salt in it is an excellent way to absorb magnesium into the body. If it's done right before bed you'll sleep better, too.

Magnesium oxide. Content is roughly around 60 percent and has stool-softening abilities. Never take more than is recommended by your doctor.

Magnesium Oils

Not all magnesium supplements come in capsule form or in Epsom salt. You can also get it as a transdermal delivery system, meaning a topical magnesium spray for your skin, which is also quite effective. In fact, topical sprays are so effective that they are often given to affixers to bring down accelerated heart rates. I know first-hand how good these topical sprays are because I've used them myself.

There's an interesting story about my first experience with magnesium sprays. I was out doing yard work and my right arm started shaking from exerting myself. My wife had an idea, went inside and came back with a spray bottle of elemental magnesium, which she then sprayed, on my arm and my stomach. Within a few minutes of rubbing it in, my tremors were gone from my arm! That's how fast the spray absorbs into your system. And it's a perfect testament to just how depleted my magnesium levels were. Point taken. Elemental magnesium has been my friend ever since.

Types of Magnesium To Stay Away From

Magnesium Oxide. You'll probably see more of this variety in your local pharmacy than any other kinds, but they pass through your system very quickly so they have a very low absorption rate.

Magnesium aspartate and glutamate. Stay away from these varieties completely. Since they are compounds made from the artificial sweetener aspartame, they actually become neurotoxins, or poison, when consumed and damage your nerve tissue.

Magnesium stearate. Avoid this version for many reasons. First, it is considered a "flow agent", which means manufacturers add it to the magnesium so that the finished product (capsules) don't stick to the machinery during production. Second, is the fact that magnesium stearate could potentially cause you intestinal distress. Third, is that magnesium stearate is made using cottonseed oil, which has it's own shady history for being unhealthy. And last, is that stearate acid suppresses a key component of your immune system.

How much do you start with? In the beginning, you'll need to test the waters to see how much your body is willing to tolerate, aptly known as your "bowel tolerance". If you immediately begin to have loose stools, you'll need to back down the dosage until you get to a comfortable amount where your stools are normal. Once you achieve a reasonable dosage that doesn't produce loose stools, you'll want to add in calcium at a 2:1 ratio for maintenance purposes until you reach the recommended level.

If you begin taking magnesium and you don't see a change in bowel movements it's probably because you're so deficient in it that your body is sucking up whatever you're giving it and utilizing it. That's a good thing because now you know firsthand just how depleted your body was. Just keep taking the magnesium and eventually your levels will come up to normal. When you start seeing a softening of your stools you'll know that it's time to cut back down to a maintenance level. Since magnesium is used so abundantly in your body it's kind of hard to get too much because any excess magnesium is excreted from your body.

Another great way to introduce magnesium is to spray it on the bottoms of your feet right before you go to bed. Not only is this a great and quick way to absorb it into your system, but it will help you sleep better. For those of us who suffer from restless leg syndrome, it does wonders for reducing them too.

Chapter 13

Things That Make Parkinson Symptoms Worse

Unlike some medical conditions whose severity have the ability to come and go based on your lifestyle or can be completely disappear (Such as diabetes), once you have Parkinson's, you have it for life. Unfortunately, there's nothing that can be done about turning back the clock. With that being said, you have to remember one very important thing:

Parkinson's does *not* completely control you: to a large extent, *you* can control Parkinson's.

Not only do I firmly believe this, but after talking with hundreds of other individuals with Parkinson's, they also agree that you can determine, again, within reason, how much this disease is going to take from you and how quickly it's going to take it. That's why the advice I'm going to be covering in this chapter is going to be of such importance because none of us want to give away any more of our abilities than we have to, any sooner than we have to.

There is still some controversy about what actually causes Parkinson's in the first place. Of course, once you have it I guess it doesn't really matter all that much how you got it, just that you got it. Even though no one can definitively point a finger at an exact cause, there are certain things that we do or that we're exposed to that have been rumored by more than one "expert" to be a possible contributing factor to someone developing Parkinson's. The bottom line is, the cleaner we can live our lives and the more of these questionable factors we can eliminate from our lives, the better off we'll be and the less this dreaded disease will take from us.

1. Excess Weight

Anytime you have excess weight, you're putting yourself at risk of developing a list of medical conditions a mile long. But for

Parkinson patients, maintaining a proper weight is of importance for an entirely different reason because carrying around excess weight affects your stability.

You can't be as agile on your feet when you're heavier and for someone who already has balance issues, having something else to throw off your stability isn't a good idea- especially when that something else can be eliminated.

Sporting extra weight can make it much more difficult for you to get in and out of chairs, beds and cars, regardless of how young or old you are simply because of how stable your posture is. It can also wear you out faster and interfere with your gait since you're being forced to overexert yourself more than you should. But the worst part of struggling to move about is the increased fear of falling.

As Parkinson's disease progresses, the muscles in our upper torso begin to tighten and shorten, instinctively pulling our frame forward causing us to begin to lose our center of gravity more and more. When you factor in the point that your head weighs between 7 and 10 pounds, leaning forward means that you're not only having to make adjustments to try to balance out your upper torso, but now you're also having to compensate for the additional weight of your head even more than usual. Even with an ideal weight, trying to stay upright is a challenge, to say the least. Adding excess weight, most prominently in the abdominal area, throws you off-balance even more and makes the situation that much worse.

2. Aluminum

Aluminum is the most commonly-used and distributed metal on the planet. Aside from its industrial uses, it's used to make cookware and a variety of food products that I'll list in a minute. But as convenient and prevalent as aluminum is, it should come with a warning label because using it still isn't worth the risks that you're subjecting your health to.

The fact is that aluminum is one of the most dangerous substances we come into contact with. This might sound a bit odd to you and even a tad dramatic, but there's tons of research to back up this fact. The point here is that our bodies have absolutely no use for aluminum at all. So any evidence of it in our body- even the smallest trace of its existence in our cells- is unwarranted and completely unnecessary.

You know as well as I do that anything that our body doesn't need or use has to be damaging or else it would be a part of our biological makeup. If you aren't aware of just how serious the issue of aluminum is you really need to pay attention to what I'm about to tell you.

It doesn't matter how you're exposed to it, whether it be from the inhalation of dust particles, tiny specs coming off of cookware or traces found in vaccinations, aluminum is just as dangerous in any form. But some of us have it much worse than others. Those who work in jobs involving any type of burning of metal (steel industry, body shops and welding, for example), are at particularly higher risks of exposure than the general public.

Like other heavy metals, once aluminum enters your body, it travels via your bloodstream until it ends up in your brain. Nothing can stop it from settling there- nothing- not even the blood-brain barrier that keeps so many other toxins away. Once it's there, it immediately begins an unrelenting all-out assault on your central nervous system. Aluminum doesn't dissipate so all you're doing is adding to the tally that accumulates.

It is well-documented that heavy metals cause toxicity of the brain with aluminum being one of the worst out of all of them. The scary part is that it's found everywhere. In fact, there's a good chance that many of the medications you routinely take right now contain aluminum- especially antacids, anti-diarrhea medications and even some pain killers. That's right, even some of your own medications contain aluminum.

When you take a closer look at health-care products, you'll find aluminum in everything from shampoo to toothpaste and even teeth-whitening products. But one of the biggest culprits for exposing us to aluminum is, believe it or not, deodorant.

Take a close look at any anti-perspirant deodorant and you'll see aluminum as one of the primary agents, if not the main ingredient. Deodorant sprays with aluminum are just as bad as roll-ons because you're not only absorbing it into your skin, but you're inhaling the vapors, too. (If you're looking to remain aluminum-free, go with plain deodorant without an antiperspirant. Most contain no aluminum).

How much of a problem is aluminum to our health? Well, autopsies performed on patients who had suffered with dementia and Alzheimer's do a very convincing job of proving the point. These patients had an average of *20 times* the accumulation of aluminum in their brains as those without dementia or Alzheimer's. Since aluminum accumulates in the brain, that's where it causes oxidative, toxic stress.

But the damage doesn't stop there. It also causes toxicity of the liver, lungs, thyroid and kidneys. This is why aluminum has been labeled everything from an "inflamer of the brain" to "a potent neurotoxin". It even manages to damage your immune system. Because of the xenoestrogenic properties of aluminum it has also been connected with cancer- specifically breast cancer.

Doctors, research establishments and health organizations all over the world collaboratively agree that aluminum is toxic to the brain. There is no question about the validity of this fact and there are no arguments from anyone disputing these claims. You won't find any because everyone is in agreement that aluminum is incredibly dangerous. Since it causes oxidation to the brain, and even though Alzheimer's is the primary concern that it has been connected to, followed by dementia, there is one other thing that people exposed to it have to worry about and that is Parkinson's.

Aluminum might very well be one of, if not, *the* contributing factor to someone developing Parkinson's disease. Even if you're not in any of the metal industries mention above, you don't take antacids and you don't use antiperspirants, you're still not out of the woods because aluminum is all around you.

Aluminum cookware. A major culprit of contamination, this makes up a vast majority of the cookware available on the market. Even going with cookware that is labeled as being "anodized metal" won't protect you because even though it doesn't have an aluminum base it's still coated in aluminum. Either way, the aluminum will eventually begin to flake off because of normal use.

Cleaning aluminum cookware is another issue. The worst thing you can do is clean your cookware with a hard scrub brush. All that does is accelerate the flaking. Initially, you'll begin to see it in tiny little specks that you might not really notice unless you're particularly looking for them. These flakes make their way into your food and, subsequently, into your brain. Even pieces of cookware touted as being "teflon coated" still contain an aluminum base. You should know that there are also ongoing questions being raised about the safety of coated cookware, too.

What's your best bet for preparing food? Glass. The only way to play it safe is to get rid of all metal cookware and replace it with glass.

Thought that was the end of the bad news? I'm afraid it isn't. You see, one of the groups of people who are most prone to aluminum concentration in the brain are those who are magnesium-deficient. Why? Because having a magnesium deficiency means that you have a lower number of enzymes strategically placed in the brain to offer protection. Aluminum does an excellent job of deactivating these protective enzymes.

Other places to be on the lookout for hidden aluminum include:

Metal cleaners. They usually contain aluminum oxides as the principle cleaning agent.

Drinking water. Many areas have aluminum in their water supplies. But wait: you say you have fluoride in your water so it must be safer to drink? After all, state and local governments wouldn't intentionally put something in your water that was bad for you, right? Wrong again. Not only does adding fluoride not help the issue, it actually makes it worse since fluoride works together with aluminum to create an unhealthy cocktail that's even more dangerous than aluminum by itself.

Applied sunscreens. Always check your sunscreen labels for aluminum. Even though there are safe options available, they aren't as readily available as the unsafe versions so you have to be diligent about what you choose. The best selection of safe sunscreens are found online.

Vaccinations. Virtually all vaccinations contain some amount of aluminum. Some even contain iron, which, when combined with aluminum, create a more toxic situation. Here are the most common aluminum-laden vaccinations: Gardasil (HPV), DTaP (diphtheria, tetanus, pertussis, pneumococcal), HiB (haemophilus influenza) and Hepatitis A and B.

Packaged foods. If food is wrapped in something with an aluminum content (such as some frozen TV dinners, frozen lasagnas, etc.), the aluminum will leech out into the food- especially when it's heated.

Pouch drinks. Specific brands are packaged in aluminum-lined containers. If you aren't sure whether the brand you see is included in this group you can either call the manufacturer or dissect one and see if you can tell by looking at it. If there's any question whatsoever, pass on it.

Processed foods. Added into many packaged, processed foods as an emulsifying agent which is used to mix several ingredients together. These include, but are not limited to, self-rising flour, cake mixes, chocolate mixes, waffles, any type of prepared dough, baking soda, non-dairy creamers and even pickles. But one of the worst offenders is processed cheeses- particularly the single-sliced types.

Additives. Be on the lookout for processed foods that list these specific additives in their ingredients list:

- Bauxite (aluminum oxide)
- E173
- E520
- E521
- E523
- E541
- E545
- E554
- E555
- E556
- E559

Chemtrails. This is the visible trail of "smoke" that is left behind in the sky by airplanes. I know there's nothing you can really do about these, but I just thought I would mention it for trivia purposes.

Aluminum foil. Of course, I saved the most offensive one for last. Using, and especially cooking with, aluminum is just asking for trouble. The worst crime of all? Cooking meats in aluminum. In one specific study conducted in 2006, it shows that when meats were cooked in aluminum foil, the percentage of aluminum levels that you're ingesting increased as follows:

- Poultry- up to *214 percent!*
- Red meats- up to *378 percent!*

One final note about cooking in aluminum: the higher the temperature and the longer the cooking times, the more contamination you experience.

Some experts argue that using aluminum foil in a cool state, such as wrapping up food to place in the refrigerator is safe. I don't know about you, but I'm not willing to risk what little brain matter I have left on an opinion. As for me, I'm cutting it out altogether.

How To Eliminate Aluminum From The Body

It isn't really practical to think that you're going to eliminate ALL of the aluminum that has built up in your system, but it is feasible to eliminate a good part of it. Here are some ways to accomplish that:

Chelation. Some will tell you that the best and most efficient way to rid your body of aluminum, as well as other metals, is through a process called chelation. Chelation involves administering a chelating agent into the body (through an IV) to "wash" out heavy metals. The agent is designed to bind to the aluminum so it can be excreted naturally. Although there have been instances where this procedure was used for other reasons, chelation should only be used for removing heavy metals from the body and should only be performed in an office setting by trained medical professionals.

But as promising as this might sound chelation is often an unfavorable option because while it does remove toxins from the body, when performed properly, it does so too quickly. That might sound a bit confusing. After all, isn't that the whole idea? Well, yes and no. Yes, you want to rid the body of toxins but if you do it too quickly, you're setting yourself up for some major backlash issues.

You see, when the body starts removing toxins *too* quickly, it puts too much of a strain on your detoxification system. It quickly becomes overloaded with toxins that have been neatly stashed away in your tissue. When you start releasing all of these hidden poisons all at once and they flood the body it's simply more than the body can withstand. Your detoxification system isn't prepared for the onslaught of toxins being released and it becomes overwhelmed. Now that you've awakened all of these poisons, they get to work doing what they do best: destroying your health. Before all of the toxins can be excreted, they do some nasty things to your body including joint pain, moodiness, irritability and even acne.

But chelation should not be your first choice for another reason. This procedure must be, and rightfully should be, performed under very tight supervision because of the inherent dangers that can occur. Possible risks include minor ones ranging from dehydration, damage to kidneys and low blood calcium to more severe reactions including neurological disorders bought on by toxicity, an increased risk of developing some types of cancer and, in some cases, even death. There are at-home chelation products available, but their sale has been banned in the U.S. due to the risks involved. For these reasons, most people choose to go a more natural route in order to deal with their heavy metal issues.

Cilantro (Chinese parsley) and chlorella. By themselves, the detoxifying properties of each one of these is impressive, but when placed together, they are even more amazing.

Cilantro

- Powerful toxin with amazing immobilizing and binding abilities
- Anti-inflammatory properties
- Anti-bacterial properties
- Promotes liver health
- Increases fiber
- Helps prevent bloating
- Reduces nausea associated with detoxing

Cilantro also has another benefit:

- contains high levels of magnesium and iron

Chlorella

- Binds well to toxins and dioxins (chemically-related pollutants that also store in your tissue)
- Contains methyl-coblolamine, which helps to repair your nervous system
- Increases glutathione levels (I'll talk more about glutathione later)
- Easily opens cell walls to allow detoxing
- Helps balance your gut bacteria.

Chlorella offers other benefits, too:

- contains the most easily-absorbed types of both vitamin B6 and B1
- helps lower your LDL, or "bad"cholesterol while raising your HDL, or "good" cholesterol
- helps your body retain more healthy fatty acids (due to alpha and lineolic acids)

- helps rebuilt nerve tissues

Mineral water. One route is to drink a specific kind of mineral water containing a high percentage of silica. There are several popular brands that you can pick up at whole food stores. The only real drawback is that they're pretty pricey.

Curcumin. The active ingredient of turmeric, curcumin can also be found in small amounts in ginger. If you go this route, you have to make sure to take it with black pepper since curcumin, by itself, is not easily absorbed and adding black pepper greatly enhances it's absorption rate.

Go organic. Anytime you can buy organic fruits and vegetables, do it. The less harmful toxins you're putting into your body from this day forward, the easier time your body will have detoxing.

Water. Anytime you are detoxing, whether it be from aluminum, heavy metals or any other type of toxins, you want to make sure you drink plenty of fresh water (not tap water since it possibly contains fluoride and you won't know if it contains aluminum).

Detoxing foods. Certain foods do a great job of naturally removing aluminum and other heavy metals from our bodies. They include:

- apples
- bentonite (clay): don't worry; this is safe to take internally
- blue-green algae
- burdock root
- carrot juice (fresh only)
- garlic
- green tea

One quick note: anytime you start a detoxing program, you want to make absolutely sure that your magnesium levels are up where they should be since magnesium opens up your arteries, allowing your body to excrete those toxins much easier.

It's never too late to eliminate aluminum from your life. Even if you already have Parkinson's and/or dementia, cutting out aluminum will only benefit you. And if you use some of these detox methods to remove the aluminum you've already collected, you could potentially slow down the damage that is occurring to your brain by it.

Chapter 14

Tests You Should Consider Having

Even after someone has received a diagnosis of Parkinson's, it doesn't mean that the testing should be over. The reality is, it's just beginning. In order to stay on top of this disease and maintain as much control over it as you can, you have to utilize everything that you have at your disposal so you know exactly what you're dealing with. Then, and only then, can you choose the most appropriate course of action for your particular situation.

Testing can be a tricky thing because even though a lot of people might offer it as a service, it doesn't mean that they necessarily know what they're doing. You don't want to go to someone just because they offer testing. You also don't want to go to someone who offers testing because it's inexpensive. This is not a time when you need to skimp. You have to also make sure that they understand the tests completely and are able to tell you what the results mean.

DaTscan

Probably the first option your neurologist may be willing to suggest for you is to perform a test known as a DaTscan. The "DaT" stands for "dopamine transporters', the levels of which are being measured for in the brain. Although previously used in Europe for over a decade, the test is fairly new to the U.S., having just been approved by the Food and Drug Administration (FDA) back in January of 2011.

The DaTscan is similar to a CaTscan and uses a contrasting agent of ioflupane iodine-123 injection to show a single-photon emission computer tomography of the brain. To put it in simpler terms, it uses a small amount of a radioactive drug to locate traces of dopamine in the brain of someone suspected of having Parkinson's.

While the test is usually helpful in determining how much dopamine levels have declined, it is *not,* and never should be, used as a test to confirm or disprove a diagnosis. That's because a DaTscan can show the same type of results for Parkinson's as it does for other types of neurodegenerative diseases, such as progressive supranuclear palsy (PSP) and multiple system atrophy (MSA), both of which retain the same types of symptoms as Parkinson's.

The test also cannot differentiate between these Parkinsonian syndromes and make a clear, exact diagnosis. This makes it impossible for a doctor to base 100 percent of their professional opinion on the outcome. So why use it? Because the results of a DaTscan are used as a way for doctors to rule out other types of diseases, such as essential tremors.

Another reason a DaTscan might be suggested is due to the extremely high number of misdiagnosed cases all over the world. According to the World Health Organization, 1 in every 4 cases of neurodegenerative movement disorders are incorrectly diagnosed. This happened to me in the beginning, just as I know it has happened to countless others before symptoms worsened and removed all doubt as to what was going on.

Possible side effects of a DaTscan are similar to those of a traditional CaTscan: dry mouth, nausea, headaches and vertigo or dizziness. In the absence of these side effects, the only discomfort you will likely experience is from the initial injection itself.

Is it necessary for someone diagnosed with Parkinson's to undergo a DaTscan? No. In fact, many doctors may mention the procedure to you, but will hesitate requesting one if you react well to medication simply because the DaTscan is merely an additional tool available at the doctor's disposal to help access the situation. Most patients choose to decline the offer of a Datscan simply based on the fact that some insurance carriers will not cover the expense because it is not considered to be a required procedure. Prices vary, but if you want to pay out-of-pocket for it, be prepared to shell out between $10,000-15,000.

But a DaTscan isn't the only tool your doctor can use to help determine what you have. There are other tests, which can help prove or disprove any questions they might have for identifying your disease. That brings us to the next thing I wish I'd known when I was first diagnosed:

Insight #10: The Benefits of Genetic Testing

Genetic Testing

Genes are the building block in every cell of our body that determines who we are. Today's new parents use genetics as a tool for gaining a little insight into what their children will be like. Not only do they determine our features, such as hair and eye color, our personality and other unique traits but they can also be used to tell us how likely we are to develop certain medical conditions, such as Parkinson's disease.

For many decades, researchers didn't believe that there was any kind of genetic connection within Parkinson's. It was believed that Parkinson's chose it's victims randomly within rhyme or reason. We now know that that isn't the case at all. Even though no one, to this day, knows of the exact cause for developing Parkinson's, nonetheless we do know that genes play a small part as to whether or not someone will develop Parkinson's disease- even if it's only in a small fraction of the cases.

The statistics might not be high, but for those who are affected by these numbers it means a great deal to understand a little bit more about how some of us came to be affected while others were spared.

Research has shown us that roughly one in every ten cases of Parkinson's can be linked back to genetics. Admittedly, that's a small amount, but for that ten percent, it serves as a caution of something important that they can make their descendants aware of. Having this knowledge won't necessarily prevent the disease from occurring, but it will give those individuals fair warning about what they might have to expect in their future.

As I mentioned earlier in the book, I had relatives that also had

Parkinson's (my father and maternal grandfather) so it didn't matter that I had already been diagnosed. I was more interested in knowing how much of an impact their disease had had on the likelihood of me having been diagnosed. The percentage of patients who have it passed down to them might only be 10 percent, but to be realistic, someone has to be that 10 percent. In this case, I was one of them.

But don't fall into a panic because even if you have a family history it doesn't mean you'll also develop Parkinson's. In certain instances, it even has the ability to skip a generation altogether. That means you can have genetic testing done, score high on the genetic likelihood of passing Parkinson's down to one of your children and they still don't end up with it.

How necessary is genetic testing for Parkinson's? This test is completely voluntary, but it will provide you with helpful information that you can then pass down to your descending family members. What's the cost? About $100. Who should have it? The guidelines say when there are at least three people in a family who develop Parkinson's, it can almost assuredly be traced back to a gene that made these select individuals more prone to the disease instead of others. My thoughts were if I had ANYONE in my immediate family who had Parkinson's, I wanted to be tested. Once I received my genetic testing results, I found out that I certainly fit that criteria and then it all started to come together and make sense.

I used the 23andme.com test kit which, even though your test results are given to you, you won't have a clue how to interpret them because they're all in technical jargon. In order to understand them you'll be referred to another site where you can upload your results and they will decipher them for you and put them into layman's terms.

My results confirmed what I already knew that I was, indeed, prone to neurological disorders from both sides of my family. Having it spelled out clearly wasn't much of a consolation for me, but it did serve as another platform to validate that I was part of that 10 percent who are genetically prone to having Parkinson's.

So far, science has pinpointed a total of 7 genes that can be directly linked to Parkinson's disease. Some of these genes apply to specific age groups while others target other factors. But don't panic just because you have genetic testing and it shows the presence of some of these genes. Even having just one of these gene mutations is still not a guarantee that you will develop Parkinson's.

Heavy Metal Testing

You might not believe that this is an issue for you, but unfortunately if you do, you would probably be wrong. That's why it's important for you to read through this section, even if you feel it doesn't apply to you.

Unless you happen to live in a plastic bubble, like it or not, we *all* have heavy metal in our bodies (aside from the metal fillings that some of us are still sporting). It might not seem possible because most of us don't really understand that much about heavy metals and what they can do to our bodies. We tend not to think about such things until such a time as they begin to show up as health issues. Well, I don't mean to alarm you but if you're reading this book, that time is *now*.

The main culprits that we should be concerned with are aluminum (which I've already covered), lead, iron, mercury and manganese. They all have two similarities:

- each of them are extremely dangerous to us and
- each one eventually targets a specific part of our bodes where it begins to do damage.

Let's cover each one of these so you can see what you're up against.

Lead

Research shows us that people who are exposed to higher-than-normal levels of lead during their lifetime are three times more likely to develop Parkinson's disease. The prevailing question is: which of us have received the most exposure?

Lead accumulates in your liver, kidneys, teeth, bones and, sadly, your brain. Any level of lead is considered to be unsafe and dangerous so don't be fooled into thinking that there is such a thing as having a "safe" level of lead in your body. As important as each of these areas of the body are concerning contamination for this segment we're going to discuss its connection to your bones. You'll understand why I chose bones in a second.

Since lead settles into your bones, the best way to measure someone's exposure is to take X-rays of specific bones using a special type of machine. The bones which are ideal for detailing this information are the kneecap and the tibia, or the stronger of the two lower leg bones (also called the shinbone).

Our bodies have the ability to renew the kneecap approximately every 8 years while renewing the tibia takes a little longer, approximately 20 years. This is important because measuring each one gives us insights to both the severity of the individual's short-term exposure rate (using data from the kneecap) versus their long-term exposure rate (using data from the tibia).

In addition to x-rays, the individual has a to be questioned about specific lifestyle choices such as their occupation and smoking. Whether or not the individual is a smoker is crucial data because studies show that even though smoking is harmful to so many areas of your health, it actually lowers your risk of developing Parkinson's disease (you just have to decide if the chance at that added insurance against Parkinson's is worth the risk or jeopardizing other areas of your health).

What researchers found was that those with higher levels of lead in the tibia were more likely to develop Parkinson's. As you might imagine, the higher the levels, the higher the risk. In fact, those with the highest levels were three times as likely to develop Parkinson's. On the other hand, researchers found little connection between high lead levels in the kneecap and Parkinson's, leading them to believe that the formation of Parkinson's is based more on chronic exposure to lead than it is for acute exposure.

Typically, lead levels are checked using blood samples, but these can be somewhat helpful they are not conclusive since lead blood samples only show short-term exposure to lead.

A good question might be: "if lead collects in the bones, how does it spur on Parkinson's, which is a degenerative *brain* disorder?" The answer is that regardless of where this heavy metal ends up, it is still classified as a neurotoxin. Our brains rely on the ability of neurotransmitters to signal neurons. Lead impedes these transmissions.

Researchers aren't exactly sure how lead alters the nerve cells located in the brain, but they do know that lead damages the signaling pathways used for transporting certain chemicals to the hippocampus that are critical for memory and learning, among other things. The hippocampus just so happens to be the area of the brain that undergoes atrophy, or a wasting away of cells due to Parkinson's.

Children exposed to excessive levels of lead experience difficulty learning and memory issues. They also tend to have an inability to focus. Interestingly enough, girls are safer from early lead exposure than boys. Scientists believe this added layer of protection can be attributed to high levels of the female hormone, estrogen. For adults, this level of lead exposure culminates as something else: degenerative brain disorders.

A common method of lead exposure is old paint. Homes built up until around the late 1940s used lead paint indoors. As old paint would begin peeling off the walls, it would sometimes find its way into the mouths of curious small children. Naturally, anyone who painted back then could expect to get some of it on their exposed skin, allowing it to seep into their pores. Other ways someone can become contaminated with lead is by drinking water through lead pipes (again, only in older buildings) and by consuming food stored in containers which were either lead-glazed or lead soldered.

Iron

We all know we need iron to help build muscles and store oxygen. It also transports oxygen from our lungs throughout our bodies. But what happens when we have too much iron in our system? Lots of bad things.

Having excessive iron buildup in your body allows for the destruction of mitochondrial, which is what turns food into energy for our cells. Excess iron also allows devastating free radicals to run wild. And just like lead, the higher the iron levels, the more apt you are to experience Parkinson's.

Ironically, iron is one of the few compounds that actually accumulates in volume as we age- even in individuals who are otherwise healthy- and the amount of accumulation is quite a lot, I might add. When you compare the newer cells of a young child to those of an older adult, you'll see that the adult has iron levels that are a whopping *ten times* as high as those of the child. Having elevated iron levels not only opens you up to certain medical issues such as heart disease and cancer, but it also plays a big part in the occurrence of neurodegenerative disorders such as Alzheimer's and Parkinson's.

The latest research to substantiate these findings was the result of a study performed at UCLA. In order for researchers to distinguish whether the accumulated iron was a product of the disease or if the iron buildup occurred due to Parkinson's, they used a highly-specialized form of an MRI, or magnetic resonance imaging. The results showed that the accumulation of iron dated back to when Parkinson's was first diagnosed, meaning that it was a cause of the disease and not a byproduct.

Men tend to have higher iron levels simply because of how a woman's iron levels become depleted during menstruation. Men also tend to develop neurodegenerative disorders at an earlier age than women. This same study further substantiates this point when it showed that women who have hysterectomies before menopause had higher levels of iron than women who entered into menopause naturally. How much higher? As high as the men's.

Here's how excess iron pollutes our system: the iron in our muscles and red blood cells only have a life expectancy of about 3 months. At that point, the cells begin to die off and some of the iron is recycled to make new red blood cells. But not all of it ends up there. The remaining residue of this iron begins to clump together and form dangerous free radicals, which then attack everything from your cells and tissue to your organs and even the foundation of who you are, your DNA.

But before you can begin to rid your body of excess iron that has the potential of doing you significant harm, you have to limit the amount of iron that you're taking in. One of the best ways to do is it to limit your consumption of red meat, which is jam-packed with iron. Also, keep a close eye on any vitamins or supplements that you're taking. Chances are, they're also concentrated with even more iron.

Once you've identified where your excessive iron intake is coming from you can go to work eliminating some of that hazardous iron. What are the best ways to accomplish this? Chelation, taking the proper supplements and consuming a adequate amount of antioxidants from the foods that you eat.

If you choose to go the supplement route, you'll want to pick up milk thistle, curcumin and quercetin. If you're also interested in making food choices to help the process along you'll want cranberry juice or pomegranate and green tea extracts, all of which supply chelation-like effects.

I first found out that I was overloaded with heavy metals from, of all places, my previous chiropractor. He saw my symptoms (this was right after I had been diagnosed) and suggested I take a heavy metal urine test to see how toxic my body was from it. The scale of the test went from 1 (no evidence of heavy metals) to 6 (high amounts of metals). Of course, mine came back a 6.

Mercury

When it comes to how toxic a heavy metal is to the body, mercury has earned a spot at the top of the list.

Everyone- especially those with Parkinson's disease- should be made aware of just how dangerous this heavy metal is, exactly what it does to your body and (here's the really scary part) how abundant it is all around us.

Mercury is toxic to both the central nervous system, which consists of the brain and nerves, and the peripheral nervous system, which are the nerves outside of the spinal cord and brain. The extent of damage that mercury inflicts on the body is unimaginable. But it doesn't just inflict damage to your body. It literally destroys your cell membranes and attacks your entire nervous system- particularly the brain. But the most interesting thing about mercury poisoning is its symptoms. Symptoms of mercury poisoning can include uncoordinated movements, speech impairment, muscle weakness, muscle atrophy, decline in cognitive skills and tremors. Any of these sound familiar?

I'm not implying that your symptoms are caused by mercury exposure but what I am saying is that if you have mercury fillings, it certainly isn't doing your Parkinson's any good.

When I say that mercury is all around us, I'm not kidding. It literally is everywhere. We just don't think about it because, as humans, if we can't see something in front of us, we tend not to ponder over it. We never think about it because it isn't a blatant poison that draws attention to itself or comes on fast and strong. Instead, mercury poisons you sloooowly.

How is mercury all around us? First, it's in the air, thanks to coal-fired power plants which supply more than half of the power used in this country. And each of these plants displaces approximately 170 pounds of mercury into the atmosphere each and every year. That's the same air that we're breathing. Put together, the total annual amount of mercury being released into the air is a staggering *51 tons*. That mercury has made it's way into our streams, lakes, oceans and particularly our seafood through evaporation and then rainfall.

The other primary place where you'll find yourself exposed to large amounts of mercury is in your mouth or, more precisely, your fillings. Otherwise known as amalgam fillings, these fillings are made up of a combination of metals including tin, silver and copper with over half of an amalgam filling being comprised of mercury. Despite warnings of how they endanger our health, their continued use releases another 30 tons of mercury into our environment on an annual basis. Although mercury has been spotlighted as being a dangerous heavy metal for decades, more than half of all practicing dentists still use them for fillings, despite the harm that they have been proven to unleash upon us. Why are they still being used? Because they're a cheap material, which saves the dentist money.

If you need an idea of just how dangerous mercury fillings are, let me put it into perspective for you: these days, we're told not to eat certain types of fish (especially ocean fish) because of their probable contamination of mercury and the health risks that we would encounter from consuming them. But just *one* filling contains approximately *one million times more* mercury than a single contaminated fish that we're told to stay away from. *One million.* And that's just in *one* filling. How many amalgam fillings do you have?

You'd think having this much mercury in our mouths would make us a lot sicker or possibly even kill us. So why doesn't it? Because it's still concentrated in your fillings. For the time being, the vast majority of it is still in place, but even so, it's still slowly being released out into your mouth on a continuous basis.

Mercury fillings have the potential of leeching out into your gums where it is absorbed into the bloodstream and eventually makes its way up into the brain. So even if your fillings appear to be intact, you're still in danger from leakage.

Here's another way to look at it: the vapors released from amalgam fillings pose the greatest amount of danger to your health. The fact that mercury fillings release vapor on a constant basis is unsettling. According to the government agency OSHA (Occupational Safety and Health Administration), the micrograms of mercury vapors that are released from your amalgam fillings can reach up to 70 percent of the air quality standards that OSHA recognizes as being unsafe. When you take into consideration that these fillings leak on a consistent basis you've now surpassed the levels of what OSHA deems as being safe.

But there's one more startling fact you should be aware of: every time you chew food, those same mercury vapors are being released into your bloodstream. And if you happen to grind your teeth or enjoy chewing gum or drinking carbonated beverages, your level of exposure can be *five times* higher than what OSHA recommends. Just imagine the combined level of contamination you're exposed to if you happen to be someone who chews gum, drinks carbonated drinks and grinds your teeth?

In my quest to try to slow down my progression of Parkinson's and avoid as many additional medical issues as possible, I decided to find out how much of a threat my mercury fillings were so I went to see a holistic dentist who specialized in removing mercury fillings (I have 2 from almost thirty years ago before mercury fillings were considered to be an issue. It was only in 2009 that the FDA upgraded the risk of amalgam fillings from low to moderate). Luckily, I was told that my fillings were small and didn't pose a high danger level right now, but they are still made from mercury and certainly aren't doing me any good to have them. It was recommended that I get them out as soon as possible.

Let me give you fair warning here. If you decide to have mercury fillings removed, this can't be done by a typical dentist because of the health risks involved. If amalgam fillings aren't properly removed by a trained professional in the right setting and under very controlled conditions, and I mean very specific, controlled conditions, then a massive majority of the mercury vapors will actually leak out into your mouth and be absorbed into your bloodstream and tissues.

There are very in-depth and precise rules in place for removing these types of fillings for a reason. You're talking about removing a poison from your body that could make you incredibly sick and cause you irreversible damage. If these vapors aren't properly captured and contained, it is a significant health risk that you do not want to expose yourself to. You do NOT want to test this notion.

How much of an improvement in your health can having your amalgam fillings removed provide? Significant enough that some European countries who have already banned the use of amalgam fillings performed studies on patients who had had their fillings removed. Over three-quarters of these patients noted a significant improvement in their health.

Manganese

Does anyone remember "leaded" gasoline? Ever wonder why it isn't around anymore?

Banned by the EPA and finally removed from the market back in 1986, lead had been added to gasoline since 1921 in an effort to reduce knocking noises in engines. Of course, when to first hit the market the promise of a quieter ride convinced many to switch over to leaded gasoline. But when refinery workers began getting sick and then dying, the government took notice and soon it was realized that lead was the cause of it.

In 1995, the government issued a waiver to allow another heavy metal to be added into gasoline in the place of lead. This metal is known as methylcyclopentadienyl manganese tricarbonyl (MMT). You probably aren't familiar with this name, but when it's pumped into a car's gas tank as part of it's fuel, it breaks down into something you will recognize: manganese. Don't worry: this is all about to become relevant.

Manganese is a mineral that is naturally found in many of the foods that we enjoy. In this instance, there is no danger to the body since excess manganese from our foods can be easily digested and removed from the body through normal excretion. It's when we are exposed to manganese from an *unnatural* source that it becomes a problem- a very big problem.

The biggest problem with manganese poisoning is that it can revert all the way back to before you were even born. If a pregnant woman is exposed to manganese, say from the exhausts of automobiles that were still using leaded gasoline, those fumes were passed directly from the pregnant mother down to the fetus via the placenta. After a baby is born, the baby still receives contamination from manganese through breast milk. This is important to note since a fetus and even an infant are not only more susceptible to manganese absorption that their adult mother, but they also aren't able to expel manganese from their bodies nearly as easily. Add this to the fact that the brains of both fetuses and infants absorbs manganese so easily and it spells trouble for a developing child.

The reason that people never make the connection between being subjected to manganese poisoning as a child and having Parkinson or even Parkinson-like symptoms as they get older is because manganese poisoning takes time. A very long time. Because of such a delayed reaction, the effects of early manganese poisoning may not present themselves until later years and the individual doesn't know to tie the two issues together.

But there's another problem. Inhaling manganese from the air is totally different than consuming it in your foods. Whereas manganese from food can be easily removed from the system through normal digestion, ridding your body of airborne manganese is another story entirely.

Airborne manganese particles are much smaller and, thus, find their way deep into your lungs where they quickly become firmly attached, making themselves virtually impossible to be removed before they are absorbed into the body.

Ironically, as we get older, our bodies become even less tolerant of the effects of manganese, just like when we were infants. Being exposed to manganese in our later years also opens Parkinson's patients up to various respiratory illnesses, including pneumonia. Although no one wants to be responsible for making the connection between manganese poisoning and pneumonia, you can't help but consider the fact that Parkinson patients are quite susceptible to developing pneumonia.

Besides affecting your lungs and your brain, manganese also attacks the testicles. Initial research involving laboratory rats shows that specimens subjected to the toxic effects of manganese early on had stunted growth of the testicles. When similar research was conducted on humans, the same results were found. The exposure to manganese also caused a significant drop in the production of testosterone, as well as fewer offspring for individuals exposed to manganese. This can be expected since almost all of a male's testosterone originates in the testicles.

The reason I purposely brought up manganese poisoning is because of the striking similarities between manganese poisoning and Parkinson's symptoms. The symptoms of manganese poisoning, called manganism, include fatigue, a reduction in motor skills and coordination, a shuffling gait, having difficulty initiating movements (freezing) and tremors. They so closely resemble those of Parkinson's that it can be very easy to mistake one for the other. This is why your doctor needs to be absolutely sure that your symptoms are a direct result of Parkinson's and not a copy-cat illness like heavy metal poisoning.

Chapter 15

A Guide To Common Parkinson Medications

Like it or not, at some point, everyone has to be placed on medication to help control their Parkinson's. While we would like to believe that these medications will help to slow down the progression of the disease, and even though there have been advancements in developing newer treatment options, there is still no clear scientific evidence to back that kind of claim concerning any Parkinson medication.

The problem with Parkinson medications is that they don't all work the same for everyone. Sometimes they work, sometimes they don't and, to our dismay, sometimes they even make the current situation even worse. There's no way to tell how someone is going to react to a medication until they give it a try. And since some of these medicines require a substantial amount of time to conform to your system, it could take weeks before you see noticeable improvement (if there is going to be any). While you're spending this time waiting to see what's going (or not going) to happen, your symptoms are still there in the foreground. This is the frustrating part of Parkinson medications.

Your doctor doesn't want to give you anything that goings to make matters worse, but how will they know what that even is? The answer is, they won't. Prescribing Parkinson medications is like a lottery. Sometimes you win and sometimes you lose.

Despite all of the tireless research being continuously conducted, the best that science has to offer us is to try to restrain the disease as much as possible using the same two-fold treatment options: (1) keep dopamine levels as high as possible, as much as possible and (2) use other means to diminish symptoms and improve your quality of life.

When it comes to Parkinson's medications, there are approximately

40 different options currently on the market with new ones being introduced all the time. Like any other category of medications, some work better than others, depending on the individual, the severity and extent of their symptoms, how long they've had Parkinson's, their overall health and any other medical concerns they may have. The decision to start you on a new medicine is not one that is taken lightly. All of these factors have to be taken into consideration before your doctor can make the decision to prescribe a new medication for you.

Despite the long list of prospective medications, the list of most-commonly used medications prescribed for Parkinson's is relatively short, a total of about 10. Unfortunately, there is no set, foolproof approach that works for dispensing Parkinson medications. It has to do more with trial-and-error.

It's also important to realize that the medications you're given early in your treatment can have a profound affect on your condition long-term so these choices have to be carefully weighed by considering all of the factors. The best example of this is Sinemet, which I will discuss in just a moment.

Before I go any further, I need to explain that as I talk about certain medications, you'll occasionally be hearing the term "non-essential" as it pertains to certain amino acids. The term non-essential means that these amino acids are made within the body so it isn't necessary for you to have to rely on getting them from food or supplements.

It's sad that as widespread as Parkinson's disease has become that there aren't more options for treating it. The most common medication used today for treating Parkinson's disease, dopamine, was originally discovered back in 1967. This shows us that while there have been some advancements in Parkinson medications, we still have a long ways to go.

There are two classes of dopamine: L-Dopa, also known as Levodopa, which is a pre-cursor to dopamine, itself, and D2 agonists, or, as they are commonly known, dopamine agonists. Since Parkinson's disease involves a loss of dopamine, the most rational solution would be to simply flood the brain with more dopamine, right? Well, unfortunately, it isn't quite that simple.

You see, when you introduce an external source of dopamine, it isn't able to cross over into the brain (I'll explain why next). But scientists have learned a way around this dilemma. They prescribe L-dopa, which is the precursor to dopamine with the intent being that it enters the brain where it's needed before it makes the conversion.

L-DOPA only works in areas where nerve terminals are already missing. Its use is extraordinarily beneficial because, unlike dopamine, L-DOPA has the ability to cross over the protective blood-brain barrier. This is important to note because this barrier, which is located in our central nervous system, works as a separation, or in layman's terms, a security system, between your blood and the extracellular fluid of your brain. This barrier is somewhat permeable, allowing certain gases, water and even specific molecules which are crucial for the proper functioning of neurons to pass through, while, at the same time, keeping out properties that have the potential of being neurotoxins. Scientists are constantly working to find ways to introduce medications that will breech this barrier.

But as promising as this sounds you're still not out of the woods. Even though we've figured out a way to introduce our own form of dopamine so it can be utilized by the brain, the next problem is just as pressing as the first one.

There are enzymes located within the central nervous system that automatically convert L-dopa over into dopamine. This all sounds great except for one huge problem: it does this conversion *before* the L-dopa has a chance to make it into the brain. Despite our best intentions, the L-dopa still isn't making it to where it needs to go in time. The way around this issue is to simultaneously prescribe another medication with the L-dopa called peripheral decarboxylase inhibitor, otherwise known as Carbidopa (more on that in a moment).

D2 agonists, or dopamine agonists, look like dopamine to the body and have the ability to mimic it when enough dopamine isn't readily available, but even as promising as all this sounds it still isn't a foolproof plan.

Taking external dopamine might seem like a logical answer to combating Parkinson's, but it's like Jack and Rose running towards the back of the ship in the movie "Titanic" as it sinks: it's only a temporary fix to a permanent problem. You see, when you introduce repeated external dosages of L-dopa, you end up having to take more and more of it in order to retain the same positive results that you received in the beginning. As time progresses, you also have to worry about more and more side effects from L-dopa- not to mention the other medications that you're likely taking in addition- or a worsening of existing side effects as the effectiveness of the L-dopa continues it's gradual decline.

Taking an external form of L-dopa is intended to counteract the loss of the brain's own natural supply of dopamine since L-dopa converts directly over to dopamine. But there's a catch: when you saturate the brain with an external source of L-dopa, you unwittingly cause your brain to become desensitized and adjust to this new level of L-dopa instead of solely relying on what the brain is supposed to be manufacturing. As time progresses, you end up having to up your dosage of L-dopa higher and higher just to achieve the same results you once experienced. This is the problem with adding external dopamine. A perfect example of this is Sinemet.

Another problem with introducing external L-dopa is once the body recognizes that dopamine is being supplied from a mystery source (your medication) it decides that it's no longer necessary to go through the chain of chemical reactions that turn the compound tyrosine into dopamine because your dopamine needs are suddenly, once again, being met. This is good news concerning dopamine, but bad news for tyrosine production because tyrosine is necessary in order to have a healthy thyroid. This is why Parkinson patients taking L-dopa often see changes in their weight without making any noticeable or radical changes in their diet or lifestyle.

Once your thyroid becomes negatively impacted, your problems continue to mount. As your thyroid function diminishes, your cortisol kicks in to compensate for the loss. Now, your stress levels will magically start to go up and you won't even know why. Also, the enzymes which control your serotonin levels are interrupted, lowering this "feel good" chemical in the brain. For these reasons, some Parkinson patients decide to opt out of taking traditional dopamine medications and choose to go a more natural route, which I will cover in Chapter 17.

Sinemet

A combination of Levodopa and Carbidopa, Sinemet is widely used because it has been proven to potentially help the largest number of Parkinson patients. The partnership of Levodopa and Carbidopa is an important one. Separately, each one plays a vital role in tampering down the effects of Parkinson's, but when placed together, they form an invaluable team.

The first half of Sinemet, Levodopa, makes it's way to the brain where it assists the nerve cells that are responsible for producing dopamine, but because of Parkinson's disease, are not capable of providing an ample supply of it. But here comes Levodopa to the rescue. Levodopa fills that deficit by becoming dopamine that can be used as a neurotransmitter by nerves throughout the body.

Dopamine is a product of a non-essential amino acid called tyrosine, which, in turn, is made from a different amino acid called phenylalanine. But the body's manufacturing process from phenylalanine to tyrosine to dopamine is slow. That's where Sinemet comes in handy because it speeds up this process for you so you're able to get your much-needed dopamine that much faster.

The second ingredient of Sinemet, Carbidopa, is added to the mix in order to enhance the effectiveness of Levodopa, which it manages to do quite well. But Carbidopa comes with an unwanted, added bonus. All of that stimulation of dopamine from Levodopa comes with the cost of causing nausea, vomiting and, in some cases, even heart arrhythmia. If that were the end of the story it would be considered a failure. Luckily, Carbidopa is able to step in and counteract those symptoms by completely alleviating, or at the very least, severely lessening those nasty side effects. In short: Levodopa turns into dopamine and makes you feel yucky while Carbidopa holds the Levodopa together until it can make it's way into the brain where it can be utilized while helping you feel better.

But, again, that convenience could end up costing you. Long-term use of Sinemet has been shown to develop into dyskinesia, restlessness and confusion. The Carbidopa found in Sinemet also works to deplete levels of tyrosine, tryptophan, B vitamins, serotonin and 5-HTP, all of which your brain just happens to need in order to help you properly maintain your balance, which is troubling since Parkinson's disease, itself, also depletes these compounds.

For these reasons, some doctors prefer to hold off on pulling Sinemet out of their medication arsenal and putting it in place until it is more of a last resort kind of choice. There are other options that can be tried first, leaving Sinemet until much later in the disease's progression when these symptoms have developed on their or when having them occur as a side effect from Sinemet won't be as noticeable.

There is also the issue of your body conforming to Sinemet's use and it losing some of its effectiveness. This forces your doctor to either increase your dosage, which will also increase any side effects from the medication, most assuredly dyskinesia or being left with no choice but to replace it with another medication entirely.

Dopamine agonists

The next common class of medications used for treating Parkinson's disease are called dopamine agonists. These medications differ from Levodopa in that while Levodopa actually converts over to dopamine, dopamine agonists simply copy or mimic the effects of missing dopamine in the brain by activating the dopamine receptor.

Since artificial dopamine usage will eventually start to wear off early and become less effective as the disease progresses and as more time passes of you taking them, you might be wondering why a doctor wouldn't just start out prescribing dopamine agonists all the time and save dopamine as a last resort. That's a good question. The answer is because while dopamine agonists are similar to dopamine, they aren't the real deal.

Taking dopamine agonists compares to buying generic instead of name-brand: you might be able to get by with doing so for awhile, but, in the end it isn't a long-term solution and you aren't going to experience the same high-quality results as you would with real dopamine. For those in the early stages of Parkinson's, though, they can work just fine until the disease starts to progress more to the point that you require something with a little more kick to it.

Examples of dopamine agonists include Requip (Ropinirole), Mirapex (Pramipexole) and the Neuro patch (Rotigotine). Even though dopamine agonists don't carry the same limited lifespan as Sinemet and, therefore, are commonly the first choice of doctors there is another trade-off since they do have the potential to cause nausea, vomiting, light-headedness, dizziness, confusion and even hallucinations.

My neurologist placed me on Mirapex, but after only two days I had to come off of it because of how it was changing my personality. My wife and children became concerned because my personality was becoming darker, I wasn't smiling or joking and I acted as if I was caught between depression and being completely void of expression. I'm not saying this would happen to you because many people find relief with Mirapex. It's just that I couldn't tolerate it.

My doctor also placed me on the Neuropatch for a few weeks, which I absolutely loved. She gave me some office samples to see how it worked for me on a trial basis before giving me a prescription. When I went to fill my prescription, I found out why I had been given samples first instead of having it filled right off the bat. Even after insurance the patch was going to cost me $610 per month. Needless to say that wasn't going to work. Again, I'm not trying to discourage anyone from trying these medications because they do an amazing job for a lot of people. I'm simply relaying my own experiences.

There are also other side effects of dopamine agonists some people encounter that you should be made aware of. These include compulsive behavior, such as gambling or shopping addictions where none previously existed before and hypersexuality. You might think that this last one would be a blessing, but it isn't what you think. In this instance I'm talking about turning that compulsion into such activities as obsessively watching online porn and becoming promiscuous.

There is no guarantee that an individual on dopamine agonists will exhibit these types of behaviors. In fact, many doctors are quick to point out that if the patient is warned in advance of what to be on the lookout for, they (along with their family's help and oversight) can usually stop these issues before they become a problem. It's when a patient isn't fairly warned about the possibilities or they choose to ignore the advice altogether and dismiss it that they can get themselves into serious trouble. The good news is that these symptoms often either improve or stop altogether once the individual stops taking these medications.

MAO-B Inhibitors

There are enzymes located in the brain that work to break down certain chemicals- including dopamine. One way to stop this attack is by way of a monoamine oxidase type-B, or MAO-B inhibitor, which slows the breakdown of dopamine, allowing more of it to survive so that it can be utilized by the brain.

There are some rumors that the popular MAO-B inhibitors Azilect and Selegilene are able to slow down and, some believe, even stop the progression of Parkinson's, but, much to everyone's dismay, those claims have not been fully substantiated and, therefore, cannot be considered reliable. For now, patients with more advanced cases of Parkinson's disease can use medications in this class in conjunction with other Parkinson's medications, the most common one being Levodopa. For those newly-diagnosed, MAO-B inhibitors offer enough assistance that they can usually be prescribed by themselves.

While some of the side effects of MAO-B inhibitors can mirror those of dopamine agonists, there is also the possibility that the patient will also experience headaches, joint pain and other body aches resembling the flu. This is a valid concern that you should be on the lookout for considering how dangerous something like pneumonia can be for someone with Parkinson's. If a patient is elderly, they may also experience hallucinations and confusion, as well.

Anticholinergics

There are certain neurotransmitters in our central and peripheral nervous systems called acetylcholine that attach themselves to the receptors in our nerve cells, causing them damage. Anticholinergics work to block this harmful action of acetylcholine. Taken with levodopa, they are especially helpful in reducing the severity of tremors. However, due to risks to your health, long-term use of this class of medications is not recommended.

Amantadine

This drug was originally introduced back in 1969 as, believe it or not, a treatment for influenza. Some years later, it was determined that amantadine could also be used in the treatment of Parkinson's disease.

There have been quite a few studies which took a closer look at the effectiveness of amantadine against the symptoms of Parkinson's. However, none of these consisted of what would be considered a large focus group, nor have any newer studies taken place recently. Like other Parkinson medications, amantadine has the ability to help some, but not everyone. It is often commonly used to help extend the effects of Sinemet. That's what it does for me. I noticed the effects immediately and have been on it ever since.

Besides the typical side effects that appear to come with just about any Parkinson's medications, one of the only real concerns for someone interested in taking amantadine is directed at anyone who has renal issues. That's because amantadine is largely excreted through the urine, quickly turning it from a helpful substance to a toxic one if it can't be removed from the body naturally.

COMT (Catechol-O-methyltransferase) inhibitors

This medication consists of dopamine, which is a molecule of the catecholamine family. Epinephrine and norepinephrine also belong to this same group. Since methyl works to stop the actions of dopamine, you need this inhibitor to stop that from happening, which they are able to accomplish. They inhibit the enzyme that targets levodopa, allowing more of it to reach the brain.

As I mentioned previously, there are many other medication options that I won't go into simply because they aren't ones that are the most commonly-prescribed. But that doesn't mean that they aren't worth investigating so don't discount them or their abilities. In the end, your doctor will be the best judge as to which ones best suit your situation and have the possibility of helping you with your symptoms.

How Doctors Make Their Selection of Medication

There are approximately 10 Parkinson medications that are prescribed a vast majority of the time. For your doctor, the trick is finding which one(s) are going to offer you the best reduction in symptoms with the least amount of side effects. But finding the answer isn't always an easy thing to do. Your doctor might start you out on a particular medication by itself and other times they may include another medication with it to be started simultaneously. It's a toss-up as to whether the first set of medications your doctor chooses will be the perfect blend or if they have to discard it and move on to something else.

As I've said before, treating Parkinson's disease is not an exact science. It's a roll of the dice trying a new medication to see if it is going to help tame your symptoms enough to warrant taking it on a continued basis. Two different people with the exact same symptoms and in the exact same stage of progression can have two completely different reactions to the same medications. This makes your doctor's job harder, but not impossible. It just requires a little patience on your part.

Anytime you start a new medication, you have to give it enough time to get into your system so you can see the real effects that it's going (or not going) to have on you. It's often a slow, arduous process that you have to be patient with, which is the most difficult part of the entire study since all you want is relief. In the end, it doesn't really matter to you what meds you end up with as long as they work.

Oftentimes, your doctor has to take a guess as to what they feel will work best for you based on their clinical observation, what symptoms you are experiencing and the severity of those symptoms. Then they have to test their theory before they know for sure. If you're one of the fortunate ones whose doctor gets the combination right the first time, congratulations. Odds are, it will take several tries before the right combination of medications are chosen.

So, how does a doctor determine which medications to prescribe? It's a gamble, really.

Let's say that you doctor lines up the 10 top Parkinson medications in front of you, in no particular order, and, for no particular reason, chooses to go with # 1 and #5 on a whim. But after a long enough trial basis, you find that there is no significant change in your symptoms. So you go back to your doctor. This time, he chooses #3 and #7. Suddenly, you start feeling better and even though your tremors are still there, they have noticeably improved and your "freezing" episodes have almost been completely resolved. Now, he has to wonder which of this last combination did the trick. Was it due to #3 or #7? It's difficult to say for sure since both are new medications so your doctor is left with only one way to find out: process of elimination.

Your doctor switches from #3 and #7 to #6 and #7 and you notice that your symptoms start getting worse again. Now, your doctor knows that in this last batch, #7 was the common factor so the one that didn't help you and actually made you worse was #6. Next, they trade #6 out to #4 and your symptoms improve dramatically. So for now, your new medications are #4 and #7, whatever those may be.

That's how they find the right combination. Later down the road, if your symptoms start reverting back to their old ways, your doctor will start swapping out medications again until a new, better working combination is found. That doesn't mean that this is the combination of meds that you'll remain on because things change, but, for now, these are the ones they're starting with to see how things go.

Is Your Medication Actually Making You *Sicker?*

Dealing with Parkinson's disease is difficult enough without having to worry about outside issues complicating the matter even further. We turn to medication not to solve the issue of Parkinson's, but to offer us a short window of relief- however generous or minuscule that relief might be.

But there are times when that relief backfires on us. It's a sick twist of irony that the very medication you're prescribed to help relieve some of your Parkinson symptoms can actually make you worse or even introduce new symptoms that you never had before. Adding dopamine is supposed to help you move better, but oftentimes, after a period of time of taking dopamine, our body begins to take this best-of-intentions a little too far and you begin to experience involuntary movements like dyskinesia.

Unfortunately, there are no Parkinson medications currently available that don't come without their own set of issues. In the end, you just have to determine if the benefits you're receiving from them outweigh the side effects that they're causing you to decide whether or not it's worth taking.

The fact that different medications affect different people to different degrees in different ways only stands to make things even more confusing. There's virtually no way to predict, with any level of accuracy, how someone is going to react- or not react- to Parkinson medications. This makes it challenging for the doctor to choose which medications to place someone on because they don't know how well it will be tolerated by your body.

The reality is that the only way to find out is through experimenting, taking one medication and seeing whether it makes things worse, better or brings on something new entirely.

Chapter 16

Natural Treatment Options For Parkinson's Disease

I've never heard of anyone with Parkinson's disease who wouldn't be willing do anything they could to slow its progression. Under normal conditions, that generally means taking medication, exercising, cleaning up their lifestyle as much as possible and hoping for the best. But what if there were other things that you could be doing outside of the normal realm of treatment that could also benefit you? Wouldn't you be willing to at least give these treatment options a try? That's where my next thing I wish I had known when I was first diagnosed comes in:

Insight #11: There may be ways to slow your progression.

There are many alternative treatment options available for Parkinson patients that have the potential of helping reduce the effects of the disease and give you a better quality of life. Notice I said "potential". There are no guarantees or else everyone would be doing them, but they are worth a shot to at least try them to see if you're one of the fortunate ones to see an improvement.

Like every other area of medicine, some of these options will make a noticeable difference and improve your symptoms while others won't offer you any change at all. But the thing is, you won't know if they have anything to offer you until you give them a chance.

The problem is that most Parkinson patients never hear about these alternative treatments unless they're either told about them by someone else who has experienced them first-hand or they stumble upon the information themselves by accident. It's rare that someone being treated for Parkinson's hears about them from their doctor. But you shouldn't take it personally because it isn't their fault and it isn't because your doctor doesn't want you to get better. It all comes down to the fact that doctors tend not to want to shy away from traditional medicine because that's all they know.

When doctors go to medical school, they are only taught current medical trends and practices. These practices are instilled in them and, of course, the doctor takes it as the one, true way to try to heal patients. They spend a great deal of time and pay a lot of money to learn and train to be doctors under these guidelines so it only makes sense that they would accept this way of thinking to pattern their practice after. Unless a doctor goes to a school that teaches alternative treatment options, they are never really exposed to this side of thinking. They never offer advice on the topic simply because they aren't equipped to do so.

Take acupuncture, for instance (which I will cover next in this chapter). There are countless individuals all over the world who have dramatically improved their health and, in some cases, even cured their ailments using nothing more than this one kind of treatment. The fact that acupuncture has been a part of Chinese medicine for thousands of years is a testament to how successful it can be. If it were a ruse then it would have been dismissed long ago as nothing more than someone selling a "snake oil" cure that had no grounded evidence of being helpful. Yet, people still use it to this day. Why? Because in certain instances, it has been proven to work.

People tend to shy away from things that they don't understand. It isn't that they fear them but rather that they don't know enough about these things to place their trust in them. If it's new and it's different then it might not work, right? But what if it did?

Acupuncture isn't new, not by a long shot, but there are masses of Parkinson patients who still have no interest in giving it a chance. That's such a shame because it really does have a lot to offer. No, it might not help everyone and it certainly won't cure Parkinson's, but it does have the potential of being able to help some people with a lot of the symptoms that come with the disease. And isn't that what we all want?

So when do you step out of your comfort zone and give alternative medicine a try? Only when you feel comfortable doing so or when you've followed the standard medical protocol from your doctor and you still feel like there might be additional help available out there that you haven't tried.

Before I go on, let me just say that I'm not suggesting that anyone abandon what their doctor is advising them to do. That is *not* what I'm recommending. You should NEVER substitute your current regimen advised by your doctor in the place of trying anything alternative- no matter how promising it is or how good it sounds. The purpose of alternative medicine is to act as a form of *additional* help- *not* as a replacement.

Acupuncture

Since I used acupuncture as my example, I'll start with it. Ask a Parkinson patient about acupuncture and they'll likely tell you it involves something to do with sticking you with tiny needles. Other than that, their interpretation of what it involves and how it works would probably be quite limited- unless the patient tends to be younger and is more open to alternative treatment options. That's not to say that older adults aren't ever willing to give acupuncture a try, but, let's face it, we do tend to get a little set in our ways as we age and prefer to stick with what we know and are familiar with. I know I do.

The name "acupuncture" comes from the Latin words "acus"

(needle) and "puncture" (to puncture). The premise of acupuncture is based on the belief that our bodies carry pathways of energy called Qi (pronounced "chee"). All of these pathways of energy, known as meridians, are connected together to form one superhighway of energy that runs throughout your entire body. The concept behind acupuncture is quite simple: these pathways of energy are essential for our bodies to maintain good health. When they are unobstructed and our energy is flowing freely, we are healthy. When they become blocked, we become sick.

Your Qi is just like water: it always chooses the path of least resistance. If there is a blockage, it never tries to fight its way through. Instead, it simply finds an easier, alternate route. But in the process, the area that is being bypassed is abandoned and suffers. When areas of the body become abandoned by energy is when symptoms begin to flare up and we become sick.

Just like water, there are areas where Qi collects. These concentrated areas of energy are called "acupuncture points". This is where the needles are inserted to relieve the obstruction and diversion of energy to allow it to once again flow to it's respected locations. By inserting a tiny needle here, the energy blockage is cleared and Qi is once again restored. The type of needles used are so precise that they are regulated by the Food and Drug Administration.

If you are leery of trying acupuncture based solely on a fear of needles you don't have to worry because the needles are so small and expertly inserted that you hardly feel anything. Instead of the typical sharp pain associated with having a needle insert into your skin, such as with an immunization, an acupuncture needle is much smaller and feels more like a slight pinch of the skin. The needle is only inserted a very small amount so there is typically no blood when it is removed, leaving behind only a tiny red dot at the insertion point.

Once the obstruction of Qi has been cleared, the needles are removed. Depending on the extent of blockage the practitioner is dealing with will determine the length of the session, but, regardless, the needles only stay in for a relatively short period of time. It usually takes more than one session to clear these blockages and occasional maintenance sessions to keep them cleared.

A recent study conducted by researchers from the University of Arizona focused on the benefits of acupuncture for Parkinson patients and what they found was not surprising. They discovered that acupuncture did, in fact, help Parkinson patients who were suffering with balance and gait issues and stride length. All of these areas saw significant improvement, with some as much as 30 percent more.

What conditions can acupuncture be used to treat in Parkinson patients? It can help with balance, digestive issues, frozen shoulder and other joint pain, stress, headaches, insomnia, fibromyalgia, back pain, stroke rehabilitation, asthma, osteoarthritis and rheumatoid arthritis and depression, just to name a few.

If you're interested in giving acupuncture a try, make sure that you go to a certified professional with the appropriate training and experience.

Acupressure

Similar to acupuncture as far as utilizing the meridians to release Qi, but differs in that the practitioner uses their fingers to apply pressure instead of inserting needles.

Dermal friction

This involves using a flat, blunt object to vigorously scrape the surface of the skin in order to increase circulation.

Massage

Having a massage not only loosens the muscles, but it increases circulation of blood to muscles and tissues while also unlocking stiff joints. Deep tissue massages are the best, but be prepared for some soreness if done properly.

Cupping

This goes along the same lines as acupuncture in that it uses small suction cups to pull blood to the surface of the skin in order to facilitate circulation. Usually performed on the back and neck, but can be placed anywhere it is believed circulation has been interrupted.

Yoga

Yoga is a legitimate exercise routine that has helped many people so don't dismiss this as some kind of woo-woo, hippy nonsense until you've heard enough about it.

Originating in India several thousand years ago, yoga is a real exercise whose benefits can't be disputed. It might look like nothing more than mild stretching and flexing, but anyone who has ever been trained in yoga will tell you that it is anything but mild. Once you get into yoga, you'll see that looks can definitely be deceiving.

The misconception concerning yoga is that you have to be extremely flexible to do it or to gain any benefits from it. That is actually backwards thinking. Doing yoga will *allow* you to become more flexible. And who wouldn't want to be more flexible? But there's so much more to it than just that. Here are some of its benefits:

Yoga teaches you how to strengthen your core. Having a firm, solid core is crucial for helping you maintain your balance, walk with less difficulty and, most importantly, help prevent falls. If your core is strong, the rest of your muscles won't have to work as hard to keep you upright and moving.

But yoga offers so many more health benefits:

- tones and strengthens muscles
- helps speed up and maintain a fat-burning metabolism
- improves your cardio health
- reduces stress
- helps control breathing
- increases flexibility
- helps you sleep better
- improves stamina and gives you more energy
- lowers blood pressure
- helps you lose or maintain a healthy weight

My wife got me started doing yoga years ago and I still enjoy it to this day. It helps me stay flexible and I sleep better. Because of some balance issues, I can't do some of the more in-depth moves where you invert your head, but there are still plenty of moves that I can do that pay off handsomely. Like the saying goes: "don't knock it till you've tried it."

Tai chi

The actual name of this ancient Chinese practice is T'ai chi ch'uan, but we know it better as Tai chi. Although this is considered to be a form of martial arts, it is best known as a stress reducer and muscle toner as well as for the enormous health benefits that it provides.

Studies have been done on the health benefits of Tai chi, with results from one of the most recent ones being published in the New England Journal of Medicine. The study, conducted by the Oregon Research Institute, followed 195 men and women who suffered from mild to moderate Parkinson's disease. I found this quite interesting.

The group was broken down into three categories: those who did Tai chi, those who did strength training and those who did only stretching. The study found that after a six-month period of exercising *only two times per week,* the group that performed Tai chi were not only stronger, but displayed better balance than either of the other groups. How much better was their balance? Two times as good as the strength training group and four times as good as the stretching group.

But that's not all: the group that performed Tai chi not only experienced fewer falls, but their rate of decline in motor controls actually *slowed down.* Impressive.

A combination of gentle exercise combined with stretching, Tai chi is a great form of exercise for everyone- particularly older adults. That's because it's based on slow, continuous movements that you perform while concentrating on proper breathing. There's nothing strenuous or overwhelming about it, yet, it still manages to give you a great workout (talk about having the best of both worlds). Each move flows into the next so the individual is kept constantly moving, but at a gentle, easy pace.

Because it's considered to be a "low impact" kind of exercise, it isn't too much for you to handle- even if you are a novice to exercise. By only placing a minimal amount of stress on your joints and muscles, it's one of the safest, yet, efficient workouts for adults who have limited capabilities.

But one of the best things about Tai chi is that once you've been trained on the proper maneuvers you can do it anywhere, at anytime and without the need for any type of equipment. Tai chi can be practiced when you're alone or with others, making it very versatile.

Alexander Technique

Never heard of it? You're not alone: most people haven't- including me. But it has proven itself to be a helpful tool for those with certain physical limitations.

The technique was developed by Frederick Matthias Alexander back in the 1800s. No, Alexander wasn't a doctor or even a scientist: he was, of all things, an actor. You heard right: an actor (stay with me because I am going somewhere with this).

Alexander noticed that when he performed, he would lose his voice. After numerous visits to doctors, he realized that there was nothing wrong with him physically so he knew that his loss had to do with something he was doing *to* himself. In other words, it had to be a bad habit or a bad practice that was causing such profound repercussions to his body that it affected his voice. Through careful observation using multiple mirrors, he realized that it all came down to a combination of displaying a poor posture and the way he hung his head slightly forward. He studied what he was doing wrong and, through trial and error, figured out how to make the necessary improvements until his voice was back to normal.

With his own success, Alexander soon realized the potential of how this self-awareness could benefit others. He began to study the habits of others and how those habits negatively impacted their lives. He found that simple, everyday practices that people were doing, largely subconsciously, was causing them pain and discomfort and limiting their abilities. Word spread quickly of his regimen and the rest, as they say, was history.

Alexander went on to publish his findings in four books and opened schools to teach his practices. There must be something to his teachings because here is a list of just a few of the people who have studied them:

- Paul Newman
- Robin Williams
- George Bernard Shaw
- John Cleese
- Michael Caine
- Hugh Jackman
- William Hurt
- Judi Dench
- Jeremy Irons
- Ben Kingsley
- Paul McCartney

Speech Therapy

As your Parkinson's disease progresses, you'll eventually begin to notice a change in your voice, affecting an average of 9 out of every 10 Parkinson patients. It will become softer, making it harder for those around you to hear what you're saying. It will come to a point where it feels like it takes all of the energy you can possibly muster just to force out a sentence- and even then it will sound faint to others.

But your limitations won't just be limited to speaking. You can have difficulty talking while simultaneously performing other tasks, taking longer to formulate an idea or statement, memory issues, chewing and even swallowing, in general. What's going on?

Like everywhere else in a Parkinson's body, your throat muscles are at the mercy of your disease. But not only does your voice box and throat muscles suffer, but also the muscles of the roof of your mouth, your tongue and even your lips. As with all other muscles, your best treatment is exercise.

As mentioned in Chapter 4, you can first suffer from either

dysphagia (difficulty swallowing) or dysarthria (difficulty speaking), and eventually it's quite likely that you'll end up with both of them, to some degree. In both of these conditions, the treatment is the same and involves learning how to retrain your voice to recover its potential. The best recommendation for accomplishing this is the Lee Silverman Voice Therapy Program (LSVT), more commonly known as LOUD.

LSVT literally teaches you how to use your voice again. Through a series of specific voice exercises, it unlocks what Parkinson's has taken away from you, giving you back the volume and teaching you how to speak slower and clearer. It also improves facial expression, which helps to better formulate your words, as well as improving your overall ability to swallow.

LSVT also offers another program called LSVT BIG. This program can be used for either physical or occupational therapy needs and specifically targets whole body movements. It's designed to help you perform your daily needs, to avoid giving into the disease and adopting a life of inactivity and to improve your balance and walking.

Frankincense oil

The medical term for it is boswellia errata, but you'll recognize it from its more common name from Biblical times. The reason this oil is so beneficial is because it focuses on one very important function of the body which is providing an ample amount of oxygen to the brain.

It isn't just your lungs that require plenty of oxygen. Your entire body relies on it. It's just that we typically only associate proper breathing with our lungs. A healthy brain is no different. If you're going to have a strong fully-functioning brain it all comes down to receiving a sufficient amount of oxygen. When the brain is receiving enough oxygen, you can think clearer, your cognitive skills are at their highest and your memory and learning capabilities are where they should be. Deprive the brain of oxygen and those areas start to diminish, cropping up as signs resembling dementia.

This type of oxygen deprivation is what pilots go through in their training. They are placed in a sealed room and the air pressure is slowly increased to simulate flying at high altitudes. Then, they are asked to perform a series of tasks that would be simple to anyone who was on the ground enjoying a proper balance of oxygen, but which become virtually impossible to those breathing a fraction of that oxygen.

When there is proper oxygenation of blood to the brain, the brain can heal itself faster and easier and it can receive, process and retain information much easier. But frankincense oil has one other unique quality and that is that it contains an important compound known as sesquiterpenes.

Sesquiterpenes have several vital roles in the body: they deliver oxygen to cells throughout the body (most specifically the brain) and they have the ability to erase and reprogram misguided information in our DNA. What does this latter part mean? It means that it is able to erase garbled information in our DNA that leaves the door open for cancer cells to thrive and flourish. I'm not saying that sesquiterpenes cure cancer, but research has shown that by unscrambling erratic DNA and because of the specific oxygen environment they create, it makes it incredibly difficult for cancer cells to form and grow. That isn't just speculation: it's been proven.

Besides allowing them to cross over the blood-brain barrier and help to balance out delicate hormones, sesquiterpenes greatly amplify the amount of available oxygen to important glands located within the brain such as the pineal and pituitary.

How do you use frankincense oil? You can either use a diffuser and benefit from it throughout the day (assuming you'll be staying within a close proximity of it) or you can choose to use it as most people do, by applying it directly to key areas of the skin.

Start by placing a few drops at the base of the neck and continuing down the spine. You can also place a couple of drops behind the ears, on the bridge of the nose, the bottom of the feet and on the inside of your wrists. All of these locations allow for easy, quick penetration into the skin and bloodstream.

Chapter 17

When Surgery Is The Answer

There may come a time when you've exhausted all of your medication options and your symptoms have progressed in severity enough that they begin to interfere too much with your normal day-to-day life. At this point, you may have to consider surgery as a possible solution. The surgery most-commonly used is called deep brain stimulation, or DBS. The reasons behind why it's so successful for so many people isn't exactly clear, but, even so, the results can't be denied.

DBS is used to decrease the severity of some of the typical symptoms of Parkinson's such as tremors, rigidity and bradykinesia. But it's also helpful in reducing some of the side effects they come with many of the Parkinson medications currently in use. The most common symptom experienced as a direct result of meds is dyskinesia, which often occurs after extensive use of L-dopa, the very medication that is intended to help you in the first place.

DBS surgery requires the placement of either a single electrode or two electrodes down into the brain where there is sufficient "misfiring" of neurons. The point is to send an electrical charge down into these gray areas to, in essence, "jolt" them into calming down. In other words, your doctor is using electrical stimulation to regulate the electrical circuits to and from your brain. The surgery has been performed for several decades and has produced some amazing results for patients, with new advancements in the technique being developed all the time.

Since DBS is actual brain surgery, you can imagine that it is not something that is lightly recommended. It is a very serious procedure that results in a life-long change. Being a last resort means that a person wants to exhaust virtually every other avenue of treatment before they can be considered for this procedure. Although there are never any guarantees that the procedure will give the patient back the level of improvement that they had hoped for, it can, at the very least, offer them a substantial improvement of symptoms. Even though it is understandably a scary notion to have someone actually drill holes into your brain, for those who have tried everything in the Parkinson's arsenal of treatment options, they are excited to give this a chance so they can experience as much relief as possible.

When a Parkinson patient becomes a candidate for DBS, there are several steps that they have to go through. First, the surgeon has to determine the exact portion of the brain where the "misfiring" is taking place. This is an exact science and one that has to be carefully studies and evaluated since there is so much riding on it and since there can be no margin for error. The doctor will use either computed tomography scanning (CatScan) or magnetic resonance imaging (MRI) to identify the exact location of the problem.

The area of the brain that is targeted for DBS depends on the type of symptoms the individual is experiencing. For example, those with classic Parkinson symptoms will usually have leads implanted in either the subthalamic nucleus or the globus pallidus areas of the brain. These areas are located deep within the brain and, in contrast to the total size of your brain, is a fairly small area to aim for so the doctor performing the surgery has to take all of that into consideration when trying to zero in on such a small target.

First, the patient is fitted with a head brace that is actually screwed into the sides of the head to prevent movement. Next, the doctor will drill into the skull and down into the brain until they reach the area that has been indicated as where the misfiring is taking place. Tiny electrodes are then inserted down into the brain until they reach these areas. The surgeon will have to test the electrodes to ensure that they are positioned correctly before the surgery can be considered a success. The only way to do that is for the patient to be awake during the entire procedure so the doctor can ask the patient pertinent questions and use their feedback to guide them. Since the brain contains no nerves, once they have penetrated the skull, there is no pain involved in the drilling or placement of the electrodes in the brain.

Once the surgeon has successfully placed the electrodes, they are connected to a small battery pack, similar to that of a pacemaker for your heart, called an implantable pulse generator, or IPG, which comes with a hand-held remote. The IPG is surgically implanted just below the collarbone and the wire which travels from the IPG to the electrode is surgically implanted just under the skin between the scalp and down the neck to the IPG. The battery of the IPG typically lasts an average of about seven years, but its lifespan can be less depending on how frequently it is turned on.

Once everything is in place, the IPG is ready to go to work. When the patient begins to experience severe tremors, they simply turn the IPG on using the remote and gauge how much electricity to send down into the brain in order to stop or, at the very least, significantly lessen the severity of their tremors. The remote can be used to increase or decrease voltage as needed. When it is not in use, such as when the patient is sleeping, it remains on standby until it is once again needed.

The success of DBS varies from patent to patient. Most notice significant improvements in their symptoms, which is why the pre-screening process is so precise. If a patient finds that they are not benefiting enough from the procedure, they can opt to have the device removed at some point down the road, but this is rarely necessary as the IPG typically does an amazing job of reducing the severity of Parkinson symptoms.

While DBS has helped many who were at the end of their road from dealing with symptoms, it is not a cure for the disease, itself, nor is it a means for slowing the progression of the disease, but rather a way of better coping with what the disease does to you.

Non-surgical DBS

Recently, there have been advancements in DBS which allow for a new type of non-surgical procedure. This procedure uses one thousand precise laser beams directed at the same area of the brain that would be targeted during a typical DBS surgery.

The patient is placed in an MRI tube, but instead of the machine only taking imaging of the brain, it directs these beams of laser down into the spots where the brain is misfiring with just enough radiation to create a change. Although it is still in the developmental phase, there have been several patients who have undergone this procedure and have experienced similar improvements to those of standard DBS surgery. There is still some questions as to how long the benefits from this treatment will last, but doctors are hopeful that, one day, the need for surgery to perform DBS will be a thing of the past.

Pallidotomy

Aptly named because this surgery targets the area of the brain that is believed to become overactive in Parkinson patients- the globus pallidus. When this area becomes over-stimulated, it causes the typical Parkinson symptoms to appear. This surgery involves permanently destroying the globus pallidus as a way of minimizing symptoms. As you can imagine, since this treatment involves the actual destruction of brain tissue, it isn't used very often.

Thalamotomy

If tremors are your only real concern then you may want to consider having a thalamotomy. Doctors believe that tremors originate in the thalamus portion of the brain, therefore, destroying part of this portion of the brain will help to alleviate this one particular symptom.

Chapter 18

Using Supplements To Treat Parkinson's

Supplements have become the rage of the fitness-crazed who are looking for any edge they can find to achieve improved health. They're everywhere and in such mass quantities and varieties that it can become dizzying just trying to sort through them all especially since you can find supplements to help with literally anything you can imagine.

The problem with the supplement industry isn't that there aren't legitimate products available to help with Parkinson's because there are some that have been tested and found to be quite beneficial. The problem lies in trying to figure out which ones *actually help* with the symptoms and which ones aren't worth their cost. Hopefully, this will answer your questions and clear up some of the confusion.

When you look at the laundry list of natural supplements you can take to help with Parkinson's, it's easy to get caught up in having to choose from so many options. It should be noted that not all of them are going to provide sufficient improvement to deem themselves as being effective. To help you make your decision, without wasting your money and your time, I've covered the main ones that have a proven track record:

1. Coenzyme Q-10 (CoQ-10). Our bodies naturally produce CoQ-10 all our lives, but as we age, those levels continue to diminish more and more. If you're a smoker, you'll run out of natural CoQ-10 even sooner. Studies have also shown that Parkinson patients automatically have lower CoQ-10 levels.

Made by incorporating specific types of yeast with fermented beets and sugar cane, CoQ-10 is usually used to promote energy and is not only used in many of the chemical actions that take place in our bodies but is also utilized by many of the body's organs. It is also an excellent antioxidant.

CoQ-10 works by manufacturing the molecule ATP, which is found in our cells. Cells require energy in order to survive and to do their job and they use mitochondria to accomplish this. Mitochondria act like "batteries", storing this energy for later use. When someone suffers from a mitochondria disorder, or from Parkinson's, their energy levels suffer. CoQ-10 steps in and helps beef up that energy deficit.

The best way to take CoQ-10 is with a meal which contains at least a little bit of fat- but not too much. The fat helps the supplement to better absurd into the bloodstream.

I'm not trying to falsely get anyone's hopes up, but there have been studies that showed test subjects which were given CoQ-10 over an extended period of time saw a reduction in the progression of their disease. This is not to say that CoQ-10 will do this for everyone, but the fact that there have been at least some test subjects who experienced a noticeable slowing of progression was good enough evidence for me to start taking it. The worst-case scenario is my progression doesn't slow down, but I have more energy and my immune system is stronger. Either way, I figure I can't lose.

2. Glutathione. Like magnesium, I can't stress the importance of glutathione enough. This is one of the most powerful antioxidants on the planet that naturally occurs in our body. Ranked as the most abundant antioxidant that we have, it is found in our liver and throughout our cells. It is so powerful and so prevalent that it has been labeled the "master antioxidant". Unfortunately, between our unhealthy lifestyles and our surroundings, we do a lot to deplete this important compound out of our system.

Glutathione not only helps to minimize the number of destructive free radicals that attempt to ravage our bodies, but it also offers so many other benefits:

- helps reduce harmful effects that contribute to premature aging
- jump-starts other antioxidants so they can be utilized

- helps with DNA repair
- fights chronic fatigue
- treats serious lung conditions
- promotes a healthy liver
- neutralizes toxins, chemicals, etc.
- helps supply the foundation for proteins
- helps with autoimmune disorders
- boosts your immune system

There are several lifestyle choices you can make which will offer a substantial benefit to your glutathione levels. One is to refrain from eating processed luncheon meats. The other is to quit smoking.

While you can go the conventional route and pop a supplement of glutathione, this typically isn't the most effective approach since most of the supplements on the market are difficult for the body to absorb. The two main exceptions to this rule are to go with a derivative of one of the main ingredients of glutathione, cysteine, which I will cover next, or alpha lipoid acid.

The first option is a pre-cursor to glutathione called N-acetyl-cysteine, known as NAC or simply cysteine. NAC is, by far, the most widely-used form of glutathione due to its effectiveness and is even widely used in hospitals. The appropriate dosage of NAC would be 600 mg taken up to three times a day.

For those who choose not to go the NAC route you also have the second option, alpha lipoid acid, which is considered by others to be the best way to up your glutathione levels because of how well it works in combination with glutathione. The recommended dosage for alpha lipoid acid is 100 mg a day.

Those individuals who are looking for the most direct dosing of glutathione tend to go the intravenous route. This allows the compound to go directly where it is needed in the body, bypassing the digestive system where a majority of it would be naturally broken down and neutralized. There are many neurologists who specialize in IV glutathione as part of their treatment options and there have been some amazing results achieved from this type of therapy.

But if you still want to get the best bang for your buck, and are looking for the most convenient option, you need to try to get your glutathione from food. The list of foods rich in glutathione are easy to remember: since one of the three amino acids that make up this compound, cysteine, has a high sulfur content, you want to look for foods that also contain a high sulfur base. These include cabbage, Brussel sprouts, kale and onions. Others that you might not associate with being rich in sulfur are walnuts and avocados.

3. L-Tyrosine. As I mentioned in a previous chapter, tyrosine is the pre-cursor to L-dopa, which turns directly into dopamine. It is made from phenylalanine, which is an essential amino acid, meaning that you must receive it through food or supplementation. Tyrosine is important because it influences the number of neurotransmitters your brain carries. Sources of tyrosine include chicken, fish, turkey, milk, cheese, yogurt, bananas, avocados, almonds and peanuts.

Tyrosine provides a wide array of advantages to your body. It

- helps in the production of neurotransmitters, specifically dopamine.
- helps fight depression.
- serves as a building block for every protein in your body.
- reduces stress by boosting epinephrine and norepinephrine levels.
- helps burn off stored fat.
- influences such mental functions as attention, alertness, mental performance and focus.
- supports organs such as the pituitary, thyroid and adrenal glands which are responsible for not only manufacturing, but also regulating important hormones.

*** **Warning:** It is recommended that the following groups of people should **NOT** take tyrosine:

- those taking L-dopa
- those taking Monoamine Oxidase Inhibitors (MAOIs) because of the possible dramatic increase in blood pressure

- those taking synthetic thyroid hormones

4. 5-HTP. Want to know why you get so sleepy after a Thanksgiving meal of turkey? Part of the reason is because of the sheer volume of food that we ingest, but part of it is also because of the series of chemical reactions that take place in your body.

The dominant ingredient in turkey, the amino acid tryptophan, is converted over into the chemical 5-HTP, which then converts over into serotonin. Serotonin, as you know, is the neurotransmitter that helps with anxiety and promotes mood and sleep, but it also helps brain cells communicate. But instead of stuffing (no pun intended) yourself with turkey all year long, you can achieve the same benefits by taking a 5-HTP supplement.

Supplements are the way to go because even though tryptophan can be found in foods, 5-HTP cannot. Besides, the amount of tryptophan you receive is minimal, at best, so you would need to indulge in quite a bit of these foods to order to receive a significant amount of 5-HTP. Ironically, Thanksgiving meals also encourage napping because some of the other foods high in tryptophan are potatoes, milk and pumpkin, all common dishes for the holiday. Chicken, collards and turnips also register high in tryptophan.

The proper dosage for 5-HTP is around 50 mg up to three times per day unless you're suffering from depression or anxiety in which case you can go up to 300 mg daily. Just be leery of high doses as they can sometimes be toxic.

6. SAMe. It's medical name is the mouthful S-Adenosylmethionine, which is why we know it better as SAMe. It can be found in virtually every bit of fluid and tissue in the body and is an important part of our immune system, but it's what it does for our brains and its chemicals that is so appealing.

SAMe not only helps to maintain our cell membranes, but it also helps manufacture and process vital brain chemicals such as melatonin, serotonin and, the all-important dopamine. It has been used to treat depression, although more studies are needed to determine just how effective it is in this area. There have also been studies where it was given to treat painful conditions such as fibromyalgia and osteoarthritis, with moderate success. However, it has shown great promise in treating cognitive issues, such as those experienced by Alzheimer's patients.

Dosages of SAMe depend on the medical condition you are targeting. For example, those with depression should take between 400-800 mg twice per day. For those with fibromyalgia, dosage is 400 mg twice a day and for osteoarthritis, the recommended dosage is 200-400 mg 2-3 times per day as needed.

As with tyrosine, those taking L-dopa should not take SAMe without clearing it with their doctor as SAMe can diminish the effect of L-dopa.

7. Micuna Pruriens. A tropical legume native to Asia and Africa, this plant has been a staple of Ayurvedic medicine for thousands of years, treating everything from snake bite to improving your libido. But it is recent research (and by recent I mean within the last few decades) that has shown promising results for reducing stress, strengthening cognitive abilities and supporting brain health. It even possesses the ability to reduce systemic redness of the brain, which contributes to brain degeneration.

The active ingredients of micuna pruriens include a substantial amount of antioxidants and something else that you'll find very appealing: L-dopa, or levodopa. It is the combination of these compounds working in tandem that give micuna pruriens its significant value.

If you're looking for an endorsement from someone famous before you try it, I have one for you. Bestselling author John Gray ("Men Are From Mars, Women Are From Venus"), developed his own regimen which contained micuna pruriens as one of the main supplements (the list of supplements that he took was quite long, so be prepared to shell out some money). Most of the items are pretty standard. The only one that you have to be careful about purchasing is the micuna pruriens because there are so many different varieties of it online and you have to make sure that the one you choose is authentic so you end up with the results you expect.

Gray, who admits to having developed "Parkinsonian symptoms" a few years ago, self-medicated using a wide variety of natural supplements in lieu of starting Carbidopa/Levodopa, which he preferred to remain off of, if at all possible. After some time, Gray claims his regimen completely eliminated his tremors and freezing.

I tried a majority of the supplements Gray listed in his YouTube video, but, unfortunately, I didn't see any significant results. But I'm just one case. That doesn't mean that others won't benefit for them. In fact, I have read of some who swear it has helped them, but to what degree I'm not sure. If you're interested, look up his short video online and see for yourself.

***As with any supplement, always talk to or doctor before starting anything new and NEVER change your medication routine without your doctor's prior approval.

Chapter 19

Important Vitamins and Nutrients Every Parkinson Patient Should Be Taking (and Why)

We've talked a lot about the importance of eating a balanced diet and how it can affect your Parkinson's. But unless you're diligent and you devote a great deal of attention into what goes in your mouth, you could still fall short on receiving what would be considered a sufficient amount of very important vitamins and nutrients that your body is crying out for.

It's hard to keep up with what we're supposed to include in our daily diets. Believe me: I get that. I have the same problem. But it doesn't solve the problem that we need to have the right mixture of the right vitamins and nutrients if we expect to feel our best. After all, we all want the most energy and the best positive outlook we can possibly manifest so we have the best chance at fighting this horrible disease.

It used to be when we wanted to boost our vitamin intake we simply popped a multi-vitamin and went on our way. But while this is certainly a better option than doing nothing at all, we all know that it isn't the ideal solution. We might not always be able- or willing- to plan out and prepare the most nutritious foods on a regular basis, but we can certainly add in what we're missing with the right supplements to make up the difference.

So, what are the most important vitamins and nutrients every Parkinson sufferer should have? There are so many, but I didn't want to bog this section down with too much information so I only chose what I think are the most important ones. This might not be a complete list, but it'll give you a good enough head start by listing the vitamin, giving signs of deficiency and their recommended dosage.

1. Vitamin B6

It should be pointed out that all members of the vitamin B family, also known as "B complex vitamins", help to convert carbs over into energy and promote a healthy liver, as well as healthy skin, eyes and hair. But lifestyle choices can undo the good that you're striving for from taking them. One example of this is that the effectiveness of all B vitamins are diminished with alcohol, something most people aren't aware of.

There have been many studies that point to the possibility of vitamin B6 cutting your risk of developing Parkinson's. I know for those of us who have already been diagnosed, that's a moot point, but even casting this fact aside there's still plenty of reasons why you need to include this in your daily plan.

Parkinson's patients should particularly take notice of vitamin B6 because of how it impacts the brain:

First, it helps in the manufacturing of neurotransmitters (specifically dopamine and serotonin and norepinephrine, which helps regulate mood) which are what gives our nerve cells the ability to communicate with one another and with the brain. As you can imagine, this is a huge benefit for those with Parkinson's. It also regulates the balance of melatonin, which is connected to your body's clock.

Second, it promotes overall healthy brain function and development.

Third, is the added level of protection this vitamin offers to the immune systems of older patients. It plays a pivotal role in the synthesizing of antibodies which we use to ward off many different diseases and helps regulate the production of red blood cells.

Third, along with vitamin B12 and folic acid, vitamin B6 helps lower harmful homocysteine levels, the non-protein amino acid that results from animal protein being broken down after it is consumed. High levels of it lead to plaque buildup in arterial walls and, subsequently, blood vessel diseases, heart attacks and strokes. The more protein you eat, the more vitamin B6 you need to counteract the breakdown of that protein.

Fourth, is how it has been linked with improving memory loss.

Signs of deficiency:

- short-term memory loss
- depression
- insomnia
- irritability
- confusion
- muscle weakness
- inflamed tongue and sore mouth

Foods high in vitamin B6:

- meat
- bananas
- carrots
- spinach
- lentils
- brown rice

Recommended dosage:

- Males (age 19-50)   - 1.3 mg
-         (age 51 and above) - 1.7 mg
- Females (age 19-50)   - 1.3 mg
-         (age 51 and above) - 1.5 mg

* Although it is possible to take too much B6, which could, in some cases, cause you issues with nerve damage and digestive discomfort, you would have to take a very high amount to warrant such a reaction, usually a daily total of around the 2,000-5,000 mg level.

2. Vitamin B12

There are many reasons why it's important for Parkinson patients to maintain proper levels of vitamin B12- especially since B12 levels continue to decline as Parkinson's disease progresses.

Vitamin B12 deficiencies cause neurological issues such as motor and cognitive decline, instability and a greater likelihood for the development of neuropathy, or nerve damage, all of which work individually to affect your mobility. Since it has been shown through testing that a large majority of Parkinson patients have a B12 deficiency, studies are now underway to determine if a prolonged deficiency contributes to a faster progression of Parkinson symptoms.

Boosting your B12 to optimum levels can lead to less brain shrinkage, increased health of the brain, spinal cord and the entire central nervous system, reduced stress and depression and provide overall protection for your entire cardiovascular system. If you suffer from fatigue, there's a really good chance that your vitamin B12 levels have plummeted. As an added bonus, it also aids in cell reproduction and helps provide a layer of protection against certain cancers.

Signs of deficiency:

Megaloblastic anemia. This is the most serious of B12 deficiencies. This is a chronic blood disorder that results in the bone marrow prematurely producing over-sized blood cells which can't be utilized by the body. As a result, the number of red blood cells available to transport oxygen throughout the body is insufficient.

Other signs of deficiency:

- fatigue and muscle weakness (shakiness)
- low blood pressure
- dips in mood

Foods high in vitamin B12:

- meat
- dairy
- eggs and cheese
- clams and mollusks

- fish- tuna, salmon, trout and haddock
- fortified grains

Warnings:

* Avoid grapefruit and grapefruit juice while taking B12.
* Some medications interact with vitamin B12 so talk to your doctor before starting a B12 regimen.

Recommended dosage:

This depends largely on your age, your overall health and how deficient you are. Talk to your doctor to determine what amount you should start with.

3. Vitamin C

Vitamin C helps provide a layer of protection for brain cells by fighting off free radicals. High levels of it have also been shown to greatly increase the production of L-dopa. Vitamin C also has a great deal to do with producing epinephrine, also known as adrenaline, which promotes blood flow by constricting blood vessels. A vital antioxidant, vitamin C targets oxidative free radicals, fights back against MPTP, a neurotoxin precursor which kills off dopamine-carrying neurons and promotes a healthy circulatory system, as well as good cell growth.

Signs of deficiency:

- fatigue
- muscle and joint pain- especially chronic
- a compromised immune system
- easily bruised
- moody/irritable

Foods high in vitamin C:

- citrus

- apples
- tomatoes
- red & yellow peppers
- broccoli
- asparagus
- pineapple
- dark, green, leafy vegetables
- mango
- papaya
- kiwi
- watermelon
- members of the berry family (strawberries, blueberries, cranberries and raspberries)

Recommended dosage:

- Males   90 mg
- Females 75 mg

Overdosing on vitamin C is hard to do. Since your body is only capable of utilizing about 250 mg of it anything else is dispelled out with your urine.

4. Vitamin D

This is a big problem because it is quite common for Parkinson patients to be deficient in vitamin D. Although vitamin D has been shown to be present in the very same regions of the brain affected by Parkinson's, there has, of yet, been no clear proof that taking vitamin D slows down the progression of the disease. However, with that being said, taking vitamin D has been shown to *delay* the onset of cognitive impairment and help to lessen the effects of depression. That's good enough reasons for me to jump on board.

While there are certain foods that contain some vitamin D, the best way to accumulate it is still with direct sunlight- approximately 20 minutes per day. If it's summer and you burn easily, break this up into two sessions.

Signs of deficiency:

- weak muscles
- porous bones (making them prone to easy fractures)

Foods high in vitamin D:

- eggs
- fish (tuna, salmon, sardines and mackerel)

Recommended dosage:

- Both males and females can safely take up to 2,000 IU per day.

5. Vitamin E

Vitamin E is so important in so many areas of your health that it's almost impossible to name them all. Most of the benefits it provides are directly related to its incredible antioxidant properties. One of the main ones is its ability to combine with oxygen, allowing it to become an important combatant to help your fight against the oxidation of cell membranes and their destruction at the hands of free radicals.

Even though the number of people in most areas who have a vitamin E deficiency is relatively low, there are still those in undeveloped countries who fit into this category. What causes such a deficiency in these people? In developed countries, it's due to their body's difficulty in absorbing fats due to certain medical conditions such as pancreatitis and other bowel diseases. In developing countries, the problem is generally a result of poor nutrition. There are also rare instances where a deficiency is caused by defective liver metabolism.

Another substantial benefit of vitamin E is that it protects your body's supply of polyunsaturated fats. Polyunsaturated fats include the invaluable omega 3 fatty acids found in some vegetable oils, as well as omega 6 which you'll get from green, leafy vegetables and fish.

Other benefits of vitamin E include how it:

- helps protect your immune system
- protects your cardiovascular system by reducing cholesterol
- protects your body's vitamin A levels from oxidative damage
- lessens your sensitive to the sun's harmful UV rays
- provides protection for the myelin coverings that surround your nerves
- helps to reduce rheumatoid arthritis pain (but not inflammation)
- may work to lower your risk of developing Alzheimer's disease (some experts are not willing to give all the credit to vitamin E)
- helps your body manufacture red blood cells
- protects the cell membranes of your lungs
- removes oxidative stress
- improves blood glucose (good news for type 2 diabetics)
- improves how insulin is utilized (more good news for type 2 diabetics)
- cuts your risk of cancer
- promotes good eye health and a vast reduction in the formation of many eye diseases, including macular degeneration and cataracts
- might help with reducing tardive dyskinesia (again, some experts aren't completely convinced that it's due to vitamin E)

Signs of deficiency:

The most common symptoms of a vitamin E deficit are nonspecific neurological disorders and hemolytic anemia, caused by an unnatural breakdown of your red blood cells. Other symptoms can include:

- leg cramps
- muscle weakness
- low libido
- dry hair/hair falling out
- gastrointestinal disorders
- diminished blood circulation
- reproduction/infertility issues

Since preventing a vitamin E deficiency is very important, you'll want to take it as an additional preventive measure instead of waiting too long and doing it out of necessity to treat an existing condition.

Foods high in vitamin E:

- asparagus
- sunflower seeds
- avocados
- dark-green leafy vegetables (kale and spinach)
- liver
- eggs
- broccoli
- sweet potatoes
- yams
- rainbow trout
- nuts (almonds, walnuts, hazelnuts)

* How you cook and/or store food can lower its level of vitamin E.

Doctors prefer that you receive as much vitamin E from the foods that you eat versus having to rely on a supplement. But for those who need an additional boost, the recommended dosage is:

- Males and females   80 mg.

*Avoid synthetic vitamin E, known under the name di-alpha-tocopherol. Since synthetic versions of vitamin E are man-made in a laboratory, our bodies tend to react differently to them. Most synthetic vitamin E is not only rejected by the body, but when it is excreted, it has a tendency to take other nutrients and minerals along with it.

** The only concern with taking too much vitamin E is that it can cause difficulty with blood clotting. This is a particularly a concern for individuals who have already been prescribed a blood thinner.

6. Folic acid

A member of the vitamin B family (vitamin B9, to be exact) and also referred to as folate, folic acid is not manufactured anywhere in the body so it is up to the individual to satisfy their requirements through foods or supplements.

Folic acid is responsible for assisting your body in not only producing new cells, but also in helping to properly maintain them. It is frequently used to fight depression and is also routinely given to pregnant women because it has such a profound effect on lowering the risk of major birth defects of the brain and spine.

Folic acid helps provide a layer of cardiovascular protection by partnering with vitamin B12 to lower homocysteine levels. It breaks down the fat in your blood called triglycerides, which is a common starting point for the development of type 2 diabetes. Folic acid has also been credited with reducing the risk of Alzheimer's disease.

Foods containing folic acid:

- liver
- fruit (specifically oranges)
- green, leafy vegetables
- beets
- broccoli
- Brussel sprouts
- dried nuts, beans and peas

Recommended dosage:

Males	400 micrograms
Females	400-600 micrograms
Pregnant	400-600 micrograms
Breastfeeding	500 micrograms

7. Zinc

Zinc helps us in so many ways that it's been said even a small deficiency in it can create severe repercussions in our bodies. Found in every tissue of the body, it's known for helping to balance our hormones, it's contribution to our immune system, it's abilities as a powerful antioxidant and how it helps maintain cardiovascular health as well as helping with the division of cells. It metabolizes melatonin, promoting good, quality sleep and helps regulate the production of neurotransmitters- specifically dopamine.

But besides all of those important functions, one of the most important roles zinc plays in the body is in the many ways it impacts insulin. Zinc attaches to insulin until it can be properly utilized as needed. It also helps insulin enter cells by binding to them and promotes cell health by reducing inflammation.

What happens when you suffer from a zinc deficiency? There are quite a few telltale symptoms, most of which you would never know to directly link to a shortage of this nutrient. Having a zinc deficiency means you can suffer from fatigue, a reduction in protein synthesis, low libido, increased effects of stress, an imbalance of red and white blood cells and accelerated aging.

How can you tell if you're lacking in zinc? Your first clue will likely appear as cravings for sweet and salty foods. But since these can also be signs of other things going on in the body, you'll need something a little more substantial in order to be able to differentiate this from other issues. I'd like to say that there are distinct symptoms that would only point to a zinc deficiency, but I'm afraid that isn't the case, either.

Other classic zinc deficiency symptoms are all over the board and include fatigue, diarrhea, a lowered immunity, ringing of the ears, a slower healing of wounds, poor memory, difficulty focusing and nerve dysfunction. As you can see, unless you know exactly what to be on the lookout for, you'll likely bypass this as a probable cause of what you're feeling and never address the real, underlying issue.

Zinc deficiency isn't just an adult problem: children suffer from it in their own ways. When a child has low zinc levels, they are more likely to have glucose intolerance, a higher sensitivity to insulin and a higher percentage of body fat, all things that can carry over into adulthood and set the stage for a boatload of lifelong medical issues.

You should also be aware that having too much zinc is just as damaging to your health as having too little. When you take in too much zinc, you risk zinc toxicity, which, like low zinc, damages your immune system. The best way to determine how much you need without needlessly jeopardizing your health is to have a zinc test conducted to let you know how much to start out on and then follow up with an additional test after several months to check your progress to make sure you're on the right path.

Foods with the highest levels of zinc:

- chicken
- lean beef
- pork
- cooked oysters
- spinach
- mushrooms
- beans
- cashews
- seeds (pumpkin, squash)

8. Nitric oxide. Nitric oxide is a molecule that is produced by our bodies to assist our cells with being able to transmit communications with one another. It improves your strength, improves your immune system, reduces inflammation and dilates arteries, thereby improving blood pressure and, pay close attention Parkinson patients, it improves sleep (that, by itself should be reason enough to try it). But one of the most important benefits it offers is to transfer information between the brain's cells to improve memory and brain function.

Nitric oxide is not a new fad. It had been ferociously studied, with more than 60,000 (that's right, 60,000) studies having been conducted on it. Best known for it's massive benefits to increasing blood flow throughout the entire body and to the entire cardiovascular system, it is what it does for the heart that deserves your full attention.

The walls of our arteries are meant to produce nitrous oxide, but plaque buildup reduces that production down to a dangerous level.

Left unattended, this leads to stroke and heart attacks. This is the reason nitroglycerin tablets are one of the first defensive measures used when someone is introduced with chest pain and heart-related symptoms because it begins to immediately replenish that much-needed nitric oxide. Nitroglycerin tablets are converted over to the powerful vasodilator, nitric oxide, where it goes to work opening arteries.

You might have heard of the supplement known as L-arginine but you probably aren't really sure what it is or how it benefits you. Well, nitric oxide is the gas produced by enzymes from the breakdown of certain amino acids called arginine. The chain reaction starts with L-arginine being converted over into L-citruline by the actions of enzymes, creating nitric oxide in the process.

The nitrous oxide/exercise connection

Exercise isn't just good for keeping you limber, stretched and flexible. And it isn't recommended just because it helps you maintain a healthy weight. The more important reason behind it is that it's the easiest way for our bodies to naturally produce nitrous oxide.

Exerting yourself, such as weight training or strenuous aerobics, like running or jogging, for example, forces your heart to pump more oxygen to your muscles. The increase in blood flow carries nitrous oxide with it (remember, nitrous oxide is already trying to settle into the walls of your arteries). The release of nitrous oxide stimulates these arteries, allowing them to open up and deliver more oxygen-enriched blood and nutrients to the body.

Why is this so important to us Parkinson patients? Because, like so many other bodily functions, age takes it's toll on our availability of nitrous oxide. Having a sedentary lifestyle, poor diet and the omnipresence of free radicals all culminate to decrease the amount of nitrous oxide that is available for the body to use.

Need more reasons to try it? How about improved recovery time after a workout, reducing fatigue when you need your workout energy the most, a more efficient burning of body fat and overall improved endurance?

So how do we combat this loss of nitrous oxide so we can reap the benefits of it? It's simple. Eat right, perform strenuous exercise, consume plenty of antioxidants to combat free radicals and take the appropriate supplements, such as L-arginine, CoQ10, vitamin C and, my personal favorite, Nitric Balance.

Foods high in nitric oxide:

- salmon
- shrimp
- watermelon
- pomegranate
- walnuts
- pistachios
- dark chocolate
- peanut butter
- kale
- spinach
- onion
- garlic
- oranges
- cranberries
- beets
- honey
- cayenne pepper

Recommended dosage:

There are no definitive guidelines concerning nitric oxide dosing so the best way to judge how much is the right amount for you is to go off of the recommendations on the container and test the waters to note if you see any improvements in your health- most notably your energy levels. The only way to find your appropriate amount is to try a small dose and see how well your system tolerates it- even if it is less than the recommended dosage. If it is too much, you'll experience diarrhea and possibility mild nausea and fatigue. If you do well, continue on that dosage.

Chapter 20

Exercise, exercise, exercise

Once you're diagnosed with Parkinson's disease it seems like exercise is all your neurologist ever talks about. Do you ever wonder why that is? Have you ever wondered why it's suddenly become so important to them to bring it up every time you see them when it might have only been previously suggested by your regular doctor occasionally in passing?

You already know that Parkinson's is a degenerative disease so it only gets worse as time goes on. You also know that eating right, taking the proper supplements, getting good, quality sleep and keeping stress down to a minimum all play a major part in the big picture of slowing down the progression of the disease and helping to keep symptoms under control. You've likely also heard that exercise is important, too, for helping fight off the attacks from Parkinson's. Well, as important as those other points are, that last one may just well be the understatement of the century.

While exercise does increase your blood calcium, which, in turn, stimulates the release of dopamine, it doesn't actually *increase* the amount of dopamine itself. Although it does nothing for the number of neurons within the brain, it does allow the brain to utilize the available dopamine much more efficiently. How? In order to understand that, you first have to understand the dopamine process.

Dopamine uses a process known as "signaling" to travel between brain cells. The longer the dopamine continues to communicate between these cells, the more control you have so the better off you are. In a perfect world, this would be an ideal situation. But this isn't an ideal world and, unfortunately, dopamine doesn't go undisturbed.

A protein complex called a dopamine transporter is constantly trying to remove this dopamine from the spaces between these brain cells, which is called the synapse. When you exercise, you decrease the amount of this protein and, as a result, the dopamine is allowed to remain in place longer, allowing you more time to reap its benefits. Exercise also gives these cells more D2 receptors, or places for the dopamine to bind to, which increases the signal strength of the dopamine that much more.

For someone with Parkinson's, exercise is not only important, it's crucial. Actually, it's not only crucial, it's vital. Okay, it's not only vital, it's life-altering. In fact, if you lumped eating right, taking supplements, getting enough sleep and managing stress all together it still wouldn't even begin to compare to the impact that exercise will have on helping suppress the symptoms of Parkinson's disease.

Of course, we're all aware of the other benefits exercise delivers, but for the time being, let's put aside how it benefits your heart, helps you manage your weight and improves your overall health. Instead, let's focus on some other physical ways it can help you manage your disease.

From a strength standpoint

As we age, we all want to keep as much of our strength as we can. But with each passing birthday, nature intervenes, playing a cruel trick and causing more lean muscle (also called skeletal muscle) to deteriorate, a condition known as sarcopenia. These lean muscles actually attach to your bones, giving them additional importance above and beyond just giving you strength by helping provide stability.

What causes sarcopenia to occur in the first place? Our muscle cells contain a group of proteins known as ryanodine receptor channel complexes. Sarcopenia occurs when calcium begins to leak from these proteins.

This gradual reduction in lean muscle mass starts when we are in our 20s, although we typically don't start to notice a change until we're in our 30s. By the time we're in our 40s and 50s, the reduction of muscle has become dramatic and quite obvious. As if that wasn't bad enough the skin that used to be tightened and supported by muscle no longer has any muscle bulk supporting it and has now turned to flab, producing the infamous bat wings on the bottom of your upper arms and flabby thighs.

By the time you hit 40, nature starts accelerating the muscle-depletion process even more. Starting around this age, you begin dropping one percent of your muscle mass *per year. You read that right: one percent for every birthday.* Imagine how much of an impact that has to have on your posture, your overall level of strength, your agility, your endurance and your balance.

But that isn't enough of a challenge so let's throw Parkinson's into the mix, the very same Parkinson's that robs your body in all of those areas, and see what happens. You're left with not only fighting off the effects of the disease, but now you're being forced to do it with more of a physical disadvantage than you had before due to a decrease in strength.

Now that you have a little clearer understanding of why retaining muscle mass is so important, you should know there are technically only two reasons why you lose muscle in the first place:

(1) getting older
(2) having a sedentary lifestyle

You might not be able to do anything about the first one but the good news is that the second one can be dramatically reversed with exercise.

From an oxygen standpoint

Your brain might only make up a mere 2 percent of your body's total weight, but it just so happens to be the largest consumer of oxygen out of all of your organs- and that's even including the lungs. Since brain cells can't store energy and since they demand a whopping 20 percent of the total blood volume in your body, the brain is always searching for oxygen to replenish its supply and provides its needs. This is where the infamous blood-brain barrier that I've discussed earlier becomes so important.

The brain is outfitted with the blood-brain barrier as a means of protection for a very good reason. That barrier is just that: a wall of protection. If blood comes into contact with brain cells (as in the case of a stroke, for example), the cells begin to die off almost immediately. Likewise, if these brain cells don't receive a sufficient amount of oxygen (a condition known as hypoxia), they suffer the same kind of fate and it happens just as quickly. While all cells require oxygen, brain cells are more sensitive to oxygen-deprivation than any other cells in the body.

Hypoxia can be brought on by any number of ways since anything that restricts oxygen to the brain qualifies. Examples of hypoxia include choking or suffocating, drowning, carbon monoxide poisoning, cardiac arrest and even trauma to the brain.

Besides the most obvious reason of keeping it alive, our brains also love oxygen because it fuels neurons. When neurons don't receive the appropriate amount of oxygen, ATP levels break down very quickly with brain cells beginning to die off at around the five minute mark. At that point, the longer the brain is deprived of oxygen, the more damage that occurs- permanent damage, that is.

Eventually, the individual loses all brain activity, hence the term "brain dead". Any significant amount of time less than that without a supply of oxygen and the individual can still survive, but will suffer irreparable brain damage because as parts of the brain are deprived of oxygen for too long, they don't simply bruise, they die off. Once this occurs, they can never be revived and the individual suffers permanent types of disability, as a result. These disabilities can include a loss of the ability to speak, loss of cognitive skills or memory, loss of use of one side of the body and even a change in behavior and personality.

The more oxygen we can feed to our neurons, the healthier they'll become and the better they'll serve our needs. Your muscles also require more oxygen when you exercise because they need that oxygen to break down the food that you've eaten so it can be turned into fuel for the body.

This is an ongoing cycle as the brain's need for oxygen remains constant and never goes away. Giving your brain oxygen is like adding wood to a fire. The more you add, the stronger it becomes. Where does all of this oxygen come from? It comes from the blood being pumped through your body. And what helps to pump more blood (and thus, more oxygen) through your body and up to your brain? An increased heart rate from exercise.

Strength training

Looking at your health from a strength standpoint, you're already at a disadvantage because you have Parkinson's and now you're at yet another disadvantage because the communications between your brain and your muscles have diminished as you have aged. That makes it doubly important to regain as much muscle as you can now before the loss becomes even greater. That's where strength training comes in.

When I say strength training, I'm not talking about bulking up like you're competing in a Mr. Universe competition (unless that's what your intentions are). Strength training refers to gaining back the lean muscle mass that you've automatically lost through the years. All you're doing is taking back what was once rightfully yours. An increase in strength is going to help you with getting up from a sitting position, endurance, walking and balance while going a long ways to reducing your risk of falls. It also burns off stress and anxiety, helps you sleep better, puts you in a better mood by releasing beneficial hormones and helps you maintain or lose weight, depending on whichever category you fit in.

You just have to remember to take things slow and easy when you first begin weight training because another wonderful obstacle that comes with aging is that your muscles have less utilization of protein and less enzyme activity. That means that your muscles won't have the ability to repair themselves as quickly and easily as they did when you were young, which makes it important to allow sufficient time between workouts for rest and recovery. You also want to listen to your body (meaning your muscles) when they're trying to discreetly tell you that you're pushing yourself a little too hard because injuring your muscles as you get older means it will take them longer to heal.

How exercise helps the brain overall

I've talked about how your brain literally shrinks as you age and how the number of new brain cells that are available to replenish the old ones goes down, too. Sounds like nothing but bad news, doesn't it? But what if I told you there was something you could do about it? There is, and it's called aerobic exercise.

When you perform aerobic activity, you're getting your heart rate elevated even more than regular exercise does which translates into the heart pumping more blood into the brain. This, in turn, means more oxygen is now available to keep the brain younger, stronger and healthier instead of being sedentary and letting it just sit there growing cobwebs as it ages.

What are some other ways exercise can help your brain?

1. It helps to balance glucose levels. Glucose (blood sugar) is made from the foods that you eat and enters your cells where it can be utilized as fuel by means of insulin. But sometimes our body resists insulin, largely due to the foods that we eat. Not only is being insulin-resistant bad for your body, but it's devastating to your brain, as well.

2. It helps fight off depression. When you exercise, your brain ups its production of dopamine, as well as endorphins and serotonin, all of which naturally make you a happier person.

3. It lowers stress. It isn't just the excess stress that has you all kinked up. That's the boring part. When you're experiencing stress, your body is unloading a higher amount of the stress hormone cortisol out into your bloodstream. And we're not talking about a small amount, either. We're talking a massive quantity here- far more than your body requires at the time. And all that excess cortisol does is age your brain for no good reason. A primary target in the

brain for this cortisol is the dentate gyrus, located within the hippocampus. This portion of the brain is responsible for creating new memories. Lower your stress levels and you lower your cortisol, which, in return, allows the formation of new nerve cells.

4. It boosts the growth of new brain cells by producing the chemical brain-derived neurotrophic factor, or BDNF. This chemical is of particular importance in the hippocampus, the portion of the brain which deals with memory and incidentally is also the part that is most prone to age-related declines in brain functions.

Focus on your core

If you despise exercise so much that you only want to get by with doing the absolute bare minimum, then the bare minimum needs to be your core. The reason you need to focus on your core is because that is what's going to help you the most in so many ways as your disease progresses. Of course, additional exercise is always better, but working on your core is always better than nothing.

When you focus on improving your core muscles, it means that you target the muscles of your abdomen, your back and your pelvis. This helps you with posture and walking- both of which, as you know all too well, are compromised by Parkinson's. Here are some other benefits of core training:

- it allows you to breathe easier
- it helps to prevent the development of lower back pain
- it helps prevent the formation of visceral or abdominal fat
- it properly distributes your weight evenly to help you maintain better balance and to prevent putting unnecessary stress on the hip and knee of a particular side of the body
- it helps you move about much easier and
- it allows you to perform physical activities with greater ease.

Qigong

I covered Tai chi in Chapter 16, but I also wanted to talk about something else that's similar to Tai chi, but a little more profound. It's called Qigong (pronounced chee gong). Like Tai chi, (which, incidentally, is derived from qigong), it has been practiced in China for thousands of years. Today, more than 70 million Chinese still practice it on a daily basis, so there has to be something beneficial to it.

The practice of qigong is divided into the three areas of medical, spiritual and martial and is rooted in two concepts: qi, which is the life force or vital energy of the body (the same qi used in acupuncture) and gong, which deals with how you manage and help your qi to grow (skill).

Qigong uses a series of specific exercises including slow, circular movements, specific postures, self-massage and focused intentions, all while concentrating on meditating and controlling your breathing. It uses many of the same basic principles as Tai chi and yoga:

- meditation
- movement
- awareness
- breathing

Studies which have been conducted using qigong exclusively as a treatment option for Parkinson's patients has shown very good results. All patients typically see a noticeable improvement with many patients seeing the severity of their symptoms *cut in half*. Besides improvements in balance and posture, qigong patients also typically see a surge in their energy levels, and sometimes even a reduction in joint pain.

Spinning

Bike riding has always been a great form of exercise and, over the years, has progressed to indoor stationary bikes. But now it has evolved into something that you're really going to like: spinning.

Spinning is still bike riding except on a grander scale that is accomplished inside. But it isn't meant to be a leisurely activity. The concept behind spinning is simple; the faster and longer you can pedal, the more it benefits your Parkinson's.

Since the revelation between spinning and improving Parkinson's was discovered a few years ago, study after study has been conducted with all the results pointing to the same conclusion. This isn't just another gimmick to try to lure you into exercise. This is a proven medical fact.

One such study conducted by researchers at the Cleveland Clinic involved individuals ages 30 to 75 with mild to moderate Parkinson's who were split into two groups. One group peddled at their own leisurely pace while the second group was forced to pedal beyond their comfort zone. MRI scans were taken at the beginning of the study, at the end and at a follow-up period four weeks afterward.

MRIs on the group that pedaled faster "found increases in task-related connectivity between the primary motor cortex and the posterior region of the brain's thalamus." In other words, the patients received results that were similar in patterns of activation to what a patient would receive during DBS, or deep brain stimulation. But that's even not the best part. Those results were still evident during the follow-up MRI *four weeks later!*

A similar study conducted by the Neuro Challenge Foundation studied participants ranging in age from 60 to 78 and saw similar results. Spinning just twice a week produced a reduction in tremors and improvements in balance, gait and even speech, not to mention more endurance.

But there was also another added bonus that researchers weren't counting on. Participants also stated that their hearing, smelling and taste that they had lost since having Parkinson's disease had returned due to reconnections in the brain. How's that for motivation?

If you're worried that you might be too old or too out of shape to start spinning, talk to your doctor. Many of the participants in both of these studies used walkers to get on and off the bikes and after awhile were able to reduce their dependency on their walkers as they continued exercising. At the very least, you could start out slow and work your way up. A word of caution: when starting out, it's probably a good idea to have someone standing by to assist you in case you experience balance issues.

Boxing

This is no longer a young person's sport. It's one of the fastest-growing Parkinson workouts around with boxing groups for patients springing up all over the country. The great thing about boxing is that you don't need experience, you don't need equipment and the results are phenomenal.

Boxing helps to build stamina, balance, strength, , flexibility, speed, agility and coordination. Parkinson patients who box declare that it provides a considerable bit of help for their symptoms, plus it's a great fat-burner.

Boxing programs geared towards Parkinson patients have programs for those who have had the disease for quite some time all the way down to novices who have ben newly-diagnosed. There's a program for you regardless of your age, your gender, your current fitness level or the severity of your symptoms.

Chapter 21

Adapting To A Life With Parkinson's Disease

I think you would agree that hearing the news that you have Parkinson's disease is certainly unsettling for anyone. Even if you suspected it, just getting validation makes you wish that it wasn't real and that you could turn back the clock and never have heard those words being uttered to you. It's the finality of knowing that this is something you're being forced to deal with for the rest of your life. Trying to adapt your life so that it can now include this horrific disease might not be something we want to have to think about, but, regardless, it still has to be done.

People accept medical change differently. Our reaction to it is based on how serious the change is, how much of an impact the change is going to have on our life, how prepared we are to accept it and how willing we are to make the necessary changes in our life to allow for as smooth of a transition as possible. Naturally, the sooner we accept the change and work towards transitioning, the better off we are. Many times, that's easier said than done.

But the problem with Parkinson's disease is the same as it is with many other degenerative diseases and that is that we simply don't completely know what to expect or when to expect it. Since Parkinson patients progress at different rates and often with different symptoms at different stages, it's hard to know what to expect so you can plan accordingly. The best way to face this enemy is to be prepared for anything it can throw at you. Preparing you for that is what I hope to do for you in this chapter.

Sexual Issues

Sooner or later, I knew I had to cover this topic so I figured I might as well do it now and get it over with. Some of the things that I'm going to talk about might be a little embarrassing, but they have to be mentioned so you'll know what to expect. Believe me, I'd rather not bring this subject up, but I know it's a major problem for many so it deserves our attention.

When you look at Quality of Life studies, it shows some disturbing statistics: the percentage of men *and* women who can expect to experience some type of sexual dysfunction due to Parkinson's can be as high as 80 percent. Even young patients aren't immune to this problem, with their percentage hovering around the 30 percent mark.

Parkinson's robs us of so much more than just our muscle control and energy. It can interfere with our sexuality. It isn't fair to have physical limitations and then to have to deal with this, too, but the good news is that there are plenty of things that you can do to help the situation- depending on what the situation is.

Decreased libido

As we age, it's not uncommon for many people to experience a lower sex drive. But Parkinson's is gracious enough to take that hindrance and amplify it even more. Isn't that just wonderful? Many patients experience a decreased libido and blame it on the disease without ever knowing why it happens or what they can do about it. They often feel embarrassed and find it difficult to talk to their doctor about it- and sometimes, even their spouse. If you happen to have any of these issues, hopefully there are some things that I'm about to share with you that will be of some help.

Since Parkinson's disease decreases the amount of dopamine, it is believed that this is just one of the reasons behind a decreased libido and even diminished sexual interest. Also, there is the fact that serotonin levels are decreased, as well, further adding to the problem. You also have to consider that some medications unfortunately list decreased libido as a very probable side effect.

Erectile dysfunction (ED)

I once heard a neurologist say, "there are three certainties for a man with Parkinson's:

1. their symptoms will get worse
2. their disease will progress
3. they will experience ED.

Not exactly subtle, is it? Now, I don't know if that could be considered accurate (at least, I hope it isn't), but, regardless, I can tell you that from a man's point of view, that it isn't very encouraging, either. It's difficult to accept the fact of a strong likelihood that men with Parkinson's will eventually have to deal with this issue, but it is what it is so we have to be prepared for it in the event that it does happen.

For a man, hearing the letters "ED" are the most dreaded letters we can imagine. It's something that we all fear and hope we never have to deal with. Erectile dysfunction (ED) is not a joking matter to the man- or the couple- who are dealing with it. In fact, it can be a life changer in so many ways- and not just sexually.

An unfortunate side effect of Parkinson's disease, ED can strike without warning. A man can feel like himself one day and the next time he wants to be intimate, BAM!, it hits him. Its natural for a man with ED to feel like he's less of a man or inferior in some way because he feels like he can't live up to his expectations- or those of his wife. It can crush a man's ego as quickly as it crushes his sex life.

But the reality is anytime you have a disease that damages the central nervous system, like Parkinson's does so well, you run the risk of experiencing ED. In order for a man to achieve and maintain an erection, the brain has to be able to send a series of nerve impulses between the spinal cord, the brain and the penis. Parkinson's disease easily interferes with these signals.

In one experimental study, it was discovered that inducing damage to the substantia nigra caused individuals to experience sexual dysfunction, further proving that there is a clear connection between the area of the brain damaged by Parkinson's and this issue.

We already know that Parkinson's disease impacts our autonomic nervous system, which is responsible for controlling both sexual function and response. But it isn't just the nervous system that you have to worry about: your manhood is being assaulted from several different directions, and all at once, no less. With Parkinson's, you not only have a compromised nervous system, but you also have a compromised muscular system and possibly even a compromised circulatory system- any one of which are areas that bring on ED. Add them all together and it spells trouble. Of course, if you already have other medical conditions like diabetes, elevated cholesterol or high blood pressure, you're now throwing gas onto a raging fire, making bad matters even worse.

Depression

Although I've already covered the topic of depression, it deserves another mention here- and for good reason. Besides embarrassment, frustration, stress and insecurity, you can understand why depression would also dominate and accompany sexual dysfunction.

Depression is one of the most common side effects bought on by sexual dysfunction because the man tends to feel helpless. Of course, the fact that depression is also one of the key symptoms that accompanies Parkinson's disease certainly doesn't help matters. But aside from Parkinson's, researchers have found that there is a clear link between depression and ED.

Studies show that the more stress a man is under, the greater the likelihood of developing ED. How close is the connection? One study, in particular, found that 82 percent of men who suffered with ED also admitted to suffering from depression.

That's not to say that every man with ED is depressed, but it does bring up a good point. Since arousal is initiated from chemical reactions in the brain and depression causes an imbalance of those very same chemicals, it shows why the two can be so closely connected. This is why you have to talk to your doctor as soon as you become aware of a problem because you might not be aware of just how much depression is affecting you.

Because of our busy lifestyles and the physical, emotional and sometimes financial challenges that Parkinson's piles upon us, stress is another common contributor to ED. It forms a vicious cycle that we find incredibly difficult to get out of because we become stressed, we suffer from ED, which brings on more stress and it continues on and on until we finally decide to seek help. Watching Parkinson's slowly rob us of our physical capabilities is one thing, but when it starts affecting us in the bedroom, it's definitely time to take action.

Treatment

Chin up, men, because there is hope. Men everywhere should know that ED doesn't have to be the end of your world because there are many treatment options available. The problem is that many suffering from it simply don't want to ask what these options are. I can understand this because if you have to ask it's an admission that there's a problem. And no man wants to have to admit that painful truth.

Men who suffer in silence with ED think they can take care of the issue on their own or that it will somehow get better without any type of medical intervention. Unfortunately, neither one of these approaches usually work.

Every man has heard of Viagra (sildenafil) and other similar medications prescribed for men with ED, but many only know them by name and not necessarily how they work or if there are any risks involved when taking them. Again, it comes down to information that they are afraid to ask, but need to be aware of.

The class of medications that Viagra falls into is called phosphordiesterase (PDE) inhibitors. There are at least 11 different variations of this enzyme found throughout the body. Viagra is one of the three medications of the PDE-5 group, which has been found to be highly concentrated in the male and female genital areas.

Besides Viagra, there are currently only two other PDE-5 medications available: Cialis (tadalafil) and Levitra (vardenafil).

Each of these medications have shown to be effective in treating ED with only a few side effects, the most common complaint being a lowering of blood pressure. But this is still a viable concern, especially for those who already experience medical issues such as autonomic nerve dysfunction or multiple system atrophy. Falls are a legitimate concern since a sudden drop in blood pressure can result in dizziness and balance issues- particularly when the individual is first standing.

There are other lesser-known medications such as Trazedone and Yohimbine, which can also be prescribed for ED. Talk to your doctor about your options and remember to **never start a medication without their advise and approval.**

A Natural Approach

If you're like me, the thought of having to add even more medications to our existing list of Parkinson meds (and possibly even other medications for other medical conditions outside of Parkinson's), is less than appealing. But there's good news. Besides prescription medications, there are many natural things that you can do that can help with ED:

1. Eat right. A balanced diet goes a long ways to preventing ED. The more you abstain from red meat, fast food and sugar and stick with fruits, vegetables and lean chicken, the more favorable your body will respond.

2. Drop the gut. It has been scientifically proven time and time again that the more abdominal (visceral) fat a man carries, the more susceptible he becomes to suffering from ED. Adding as little as 10 inches to your waist can increase your chances of ED by 50 percent.

3. Exercise. The more you move, the more you increase blood circulation throughout your body, which means the more nitrous oxide your body is producing. And improving the amount of nitrous oxide in your blood just happens to be exactly how Viagra works. The supplement ginseng is also believed to improve nitrous oxide supplies.

4. Weight training. Weight training or weight-bearing types of exercises causes a man's body to produce more testosterone, a building block for preventing ED.

5. Cut your alcohol consumption. Alcohol acts as a depressant in every system in your body- including the central nervous system.

6. Stop smoking. It restricts blood vessels and major arteries.

7. Adjust your sleep. Not getting sufficient sleep disrupts hormone secretion- namely cortisol (causing abnormally high amounts of it to be released) and testosterone (causing abnormally low amounts of it to be released).

8. Check your meds. ED is a common side effect of many.

Setting up your home for a Parkinson's patient

More than likely, by the time you receive your diagnosis, you've already begun to experience some changes in your physical abilities. For the moment, these might be mild and unobtrusive, but you never know how your disease will progress so it's better to be well-prepared while you still have your abilities than to try to make the necessary changes down the road when you might not be up for the task.

Before you get started, you need to go from room to room throughout the entire house and visually inventory all of its contents so you don't take a chance of missing something. Imagine the patient being in their most delicate state and what they'll need in the way of assistance in their surroundings so you have an idea of what to prepare for. Make notes of what you'll need to fix, what will need to be replaced and what will need to be removed completely. Once you've done this, the transformation can begin.

General home safety

1. Start out small. You don't have to completely reorganize your entire household right off the bat. Start with simple things (or areas with the highest amount of use) and add more things as they become necessary.

2. Adjust furniture accordingly. You want to make clear pathways through all the areas of your home. The fewer obstacles that are in your way, the less you'll have to maneuver around them to get places. Straight shots through rooms are best so if you have too much furniture that won't allow you to move things to create a safe, straight walkway, consider getting rid of a few things so it won't become a walking hazard.

Get rid of pieces that are unstable, such as rocking chairs since you might have to grab onto it in a hurry and make sure all of your furniture is high enough and sturdy enough for you to push yourself up off of. You also want to refrain from having anything that swivels (chair, some recliners) or collapses (TV tray).

3. Secure all rugs. All rugs that lay on any type of smooth flooring (wood, laminate, vinyl or tile), should be secured with double-sided tape. If a rug is overly thick and plush and requires you to raise your foot, even slightly, to step up onto it, get rid of it. Remove all small rugs as they are too hard to keep in place.

4. Stabilize stairs. Both indoor and outdoor stairs need to have secure handrails and all steps need to have some type of sufficient cover on them to avoid slipping. For concrete outdoor steps, you can get non-slip paint or peel-and-stick pads. For wooden indoor steps, consider securing carpet strips directly to the wood.

If you use a cane or walker, have one at both the top and bottom of stairs to avoid having to carry them up and down.

5. Access to phones. Ensure easy access to either a cordless phone or a cell phone no matter where you are in your home.

6. Smoke alarms. Have enough smoke alarms throughout the house

that you can be assured to hear them no matter where you are or what you're doing.

7. Night lights. Position night lights in hallways and especially in the bathroom to accommodate walking around at night. There are inexpensive electroluminescent lights that stay plugged in all the time, use approximately .02 cents worth of energy annually, don't require a bulb, never get hot and have a lifetime illumination guarantee so there should be no reason not to have them in place.

8. Shower or bathtub seat. You'll want an elevated platform for either.

9. Get a handheld shower nozzle with a long enough hose that it can be used when seated.

10. Install shower/tub/toilet hand rails and non-skid bath mats.

11. Make sure there is a great non-slip mat outside your tub/shower.

12. Use extra-large, extra-absorbent towels that require minimal exertion.

14. Beware of glass doors. If you have glass exterior doors on your home you might want to replace them with something that won't give and shatter if someone falls into them. This is especially true of sliding glass doors.

15. Remove glass-top tables. Any coffee/end tables with glass on them need to go.

16. Trade out your toilet. You'll want to swap out your standard toilet for one with a higher seat.

17. Step-in tubs. These are a little pricey, but invaluable if you can work it into your budget.

18. Avoid soap bars. Use soap-on-a-rope, back brushes, liquid soap or sponges with soap.

19. Have enough lights. Make sure all rooms are well-lit. You might even want to invest in some timers so you're not forced to get up at inopportune times to turn them on or off and so you're not constantly turning lights on and off as you venture through your home. Motion-activated lights are always the best choice.

20. Watch for floor transitions. If you have a floor tradition between rooms you'll want to install a hand rail for assistance.

21. Remove all cords. Make sure all light and extension cords are out of the way.

22. Check your doors. Make sure all doors the patient will have access to open and close without any obstructions.

23. Inspect all door knobs. Make sure all doorknobs turn and open easily without a lot of effort.

24. Check your carpet. If you have carpet, carefully inspect it for frays or places where it has bunched up. Also check where the carpet transitions to a different type of flooring.

25. Outdoor walkways. Make sure all walkways are clear, well-lit and wide enough. Sidewalks and driveways should be patched with a rough, finished surface for better traction when walking.

26. Fire extinguishers. Have enough of them on-hand on every floor.

27. Plan out ample time to rest throughout the day. Your disease (particularly your tremors) will let you know if you've overdone it.

28. Don't overload yourself. If you only expect realistic goals, you won't set yourself up for disappointment and disaster.

29. Don't schedule too much around medication time. It takes a Parkinson patient some time to be back "on" after their medication has worn off.

30. Listen to your doctor. You might feel up to a challenge, but don't take on too much until you've been cleared to do so by your doctor.

31. Stairs. If your home has stairs, ensure that hand rails are secure and steps are sturdy and do not have a slipping hazard.

32. If juggling house keys is an issue, consider having a keypad installed on your outside doors.

33. If typing on a keyboard becomes too difficult due to hand tremors, try using voice-activated software that types your words out for you. Initially, you'll have to train the software to recognize your particular voice, but once you do, all that's left is to occasionally correct misspelled words. It's also helpful if you're not a great speller.

Adapting a Kitchen For Parkinson's

1. Keep preparation knives in a storage block- no open blades.

2. Use slow cookers as often as possible. They require less preparation and less attention devoted to cooking.

3. Keep meals simple. Multi-tasking does not go well with Parkinson's.

4. Cook large batches of food at once, separate and either refrigerate or freeze the rest so you won't have to cook as often.

5. Use the back burners on stoves as much as possible.

6. Buy cut-resistant gloves for preparing food.

7. Organize cabinets so larger, heavier cooking pots and pans are at waist-level to prevent having to reach up or bend over to retrieve them.

8. Buy utensils that have larger handles with firmer grips.

9. Place your plate on a non-skid mat.

10. Use a cutting board with a fixed, hinged knife blade attached for more stability.

11. Have a long-handle grabber to reach items up on shelves.

12. Arrange cabinets so commonly-used cookware is closest to the stove.

13. Install handles on cabinets versus knobs, which are harder to grab.

14. Replace manual gadgets with ones that are electric or battery-operated.

15. Consider buying a ULU knife. Instead of the standard long handle at the opposite end of the blade, the handle is rounded and on top, offering you a much more secure grip and more leverage when cutting.

16. If you're stuck on using your large knives and other hand utensils attach some rubber gripping onto the handles. Can be purchased at any hardware store

17. Have a lazy Susan in the middle of the eating table for smaller frequently-used items to prevent having to go back and forth during every meal.

Adapting a Bedroom For Parkinson's

Since we spend a third of our lives in this room it only makes sense that it comply with our individual needs- especially since you can likely expect that percentage to go up even more as your Parkinson's progresses.

1. Check bed height. Bed height should allow the individual's feet to touch the floor when they are seated on the side.

2. Mattress should be firm enough to assist the patient with turning over during sleep and also to help them when getting up from the side to stand. If necessary, install a bed pole or half railing.

3. Use an rolling over-the-bed tray so the patient doesn't have to leave their bed to eat if they aren't feeling well.

4. Remove top sheet, which can easily become tangled around patient during sleep.

5. Using satin sheets and pajamas helps patients turn over in the bed with less effort.

6. Bedroom should be as quiet and soothing as possible.

7. Have plenty of night lighting from bed to bathroom. You might even want to spring for some glow-in-the-dark tape so you can put small strips of it on the floor to help guide them back and forth during the night.

8. Check flooring to ensure it isn't slippery. Bathroom tile should be covered to avoid falls and transitions from carpet to tile checked.

9. Hanging clothes need to be at a comfortable height to prevent having to reach up or bend over to retrieve them.

10. Think about investing in sink faucets with "on/off" touch technology.

Personal safety

1. Do as much getting ready while sitting down as possible. The less time you require yourself to stand, the less likely you are to become tired and overdo it.

2. Do all of your personal grooming while seated.

3. If buttons are still a problem, leave most of the shirt buttoned and slide them on and off over your head.

4. If buttons are next to impossible, avoid them altogether. Go for velcro or elastic, instead.

5. Use wraparound clothing instead of pullovers, whenever possible.

6. If you have to wear something with a zipper or buttons, make sure they're large enough for you to manage easily.

7. Long-handled shoehorns and sock-donners are a necessity.

Chapter 22

Parkinson's Gadgets

As your Parkinson's progresses, you will likely begin to see your abilities become somewhat limited. The things that you could once do might now cause you to incur a certain bit of difficulty. It doesn't mean that you won't be able to perform your same activities, however, you will likely need some assistance with them. There is an entire line of products available to allow you to perform these activities with as little effort as possible. Although this isn't a complete list (because it would be virtually impossible to cover everything that's available) it will serve as a good starting point.

1. Cell phone apps. Since we've become a society so dependent on our cell phones, why shouldn't we utilize all of the available apps we can that are related to maintaining our Parkinson's?

There are online puzzles designed to help keep your brain sharp and alert. Twitter is a way to keep people in constant contact with others while working your mind and the dexterity of your fingers. There are also medication trackers which are an invaluable tool to help keep track of your medications and, one of my favorites, a "charity miles" app which raises money for the charity of your choice each time you exercise. You can also buy apps that actually measure the severity of your tremors using your smartphone's sensors.

2. Glasses. How about a cup with a rotating handle that doesn't require you to lift your arm too high or tilt your head backwards in order to drink from it? The handle swivels, allowing the individual to maintain a constant positioning of the arm so they can use their free hand to tilt the bottom of the glass as needed for better stabilization.

3. Double-handled glasses can also be handy, allowing you to hold a cup with both hands at once.

4. Straws. No, these aren't your typical straws. These are specially designed to handle hot liquids, a problem that needs resolving for those with tremors.

5. Extra-long drinking straws. Something as simple as extra-long straws will prevent a Parkinson patient from having to pick up a glass in order to get a drink.

6. Having a cup with a lid not only keeps your drink from spilling, but it also holds a straw firmly in place.

7. Large grip utensils. The more handle we have to hold onto, the more stable our grip becomes. These come in a variety of shapes and sizes depending on your needs.

8. Utensils with straps. The utensil sits in a pocket of the strap, which slides over the palm of your hand so you don't have to rely on steady hands to feed yourself.

9. Swivel dinner trays. This allows you to eat whatever you want without having to handle plates of food while you're sitting or standing. Some models even come with rollers so you can place your food on them and roll the cart into the kitchen or out to where you wish to eat.

10. Scoop plates. These look like ordinary plates but with one exception: one side has a short rim with which to trap food so you can corral it onto a fork or spoon instead of having it slide off of the plate.

11. Shoes. These can be one of the more challenging things about getting dressed. At a certain point, laces become out of the question and even pulling slippers on can be a chore. Now, you have shoes that have a velcro flap over the top so they can be loosened and tightened without struggling to get them on or off.

12. Weighted writing sleeve. Designed to fit most pens or pencils, this holder helps stabilize your handwriting by forcing you to use your hand and arm muscles just enough to make contact with what

you're writing. No more having to bear down to keep the pen in contact with the writing surface.

13. Blanket supports. A small frame that fits under your cover next to your feet. It slightly elevates the cover off of your feet just enough so you can turn over in the bed much easier without getting tangled in the weight of the covers.

14. Auto handy-bar. Known by different names, this small, but sturdy hand-held bracket easily fits in your car's door striker just inside the door frame while the door is open. Slip the handy-bar into place and it gives you leverage to stand up or sit down in the car with ease. These usually have a weight limit of around of 300 pounds, but are still small enough to store in your glove compartment until needed.

15. Electric can openers, scissors and peelers go without saying.

16. Laser cane/walker. Places a small beam in front of you in your path to encourage your brain to become unfrozen. Studies have shown laser beams to be very beneficial in helping people to start moving again after a freezing episode.

17. Replace buttons on shirts with velcro. You can still leave the buttons attached for visual purposes, but the velcro will allow the patient to easily dress or undress simply by pulling on the sides of the opening.

18. Zippers. Zippers are an easy alternative to buttons as long as you can still manipulate them. Try connecting a large loop on the end of the zipper to give the patient more to hold onto.

19. Electric toothbrushes. Worth their weight in gold.

20. Phone amplifiers. These come in handy when your voice starts to weaken or become more quiet.

21. Pill sorters. I have one that has every day of the month broken down into four doses per day *and* has an alarm that alerts me if I'm

about to run late on taking my meds. The individual trays can be removed and taken with you if you going to be away from your home for an extended period of time.

22. Contact lens holders. I use these (new ones only, of course) to hold two doses of medicines while I'm running errands. They're small, discreet and can easily fit in your pocket or a purse.

23. Invest in eating utensils with a built-in stabilizer to reduce tremors while you eat. Some models can cut down hand tremors by as much as 70 percent.

Chapter 23

Tips For Parkinson Caregivers

Seeing a loved one suffer with the challenges of Parkinson's disease can be hard to watch, but it's certainly better than having them try to go down that long, disruptive road alone. Even if you don't have a spouse who can assist you with your everyday tasks, there are always friends, other family members and even certified professionals who are standing by to assist you whenever you need help. All we need to do is ask.

Those who take on the role as a Parkinson's caregiver deserve the utmost of respect. They also deserve our attention since they're giving so much of themselves. Below I've listed some tips that they can use to hopefully help make their role a little bit easier.

1. Put medications on "auto-fill". Most pharmacies will automatically fill your prescriptions so you don't risk running out of them (I would say at inopportune times, but anytime you run out of your meds is an inopportune time).

2. Keep things lively. As someone with Parkinson's, I can tell you first-hand that the last thing I want is for everyone around me to feel as if they have to walk on eggshells or pamper me. This horrible disease is already trying to rob us of our strength, our faculties and our dignity. We can't let it take our spirit, too.

3. Plan out activities for the Parkinson patient. Don't let them stay at home so they can sit around and dwell on what's happening to their health. All that will accomplish is to make things progress that much faster.

4. Keep an eye on the patient's well-being. Are they quieter than usual? Are they less interested in doing things together? Do you feel as close to them as you did before the disease hit? As a caregiver, you'll likely be the first one to witness these changes, how quickly

they come on, how severe they are and if they appear to be something that is going to cause a long-lasting effect to their personality and their well-being.

5. Be on the lookout for changes in mood. This is different than the previous entry because it deals strictly with depression. The disease is bad enough for ushering in depression, but medications can also cause this- not to mention a physical setback or discouraging news from a doctor's appointment.

6. Know who to go to for specific help. Besides your neurologist (and/or movement disorder specialist), you have a host of other professionals who all have something to contribute to your loved one's care. Take advantage of their services so your loved one can get the best level of care from the greatest number of people who are specifically trained to offer them a better quality of life.

7. Don't neglect yourself. You can easily become so wrapped up in taking on the role of caregiver that you forget to look out for ourselves. You aren't going to do anyone any good if you let yourself fall apart. This doesn't mean that you can't have a bad day- everybody has those- and, given the circumstances, it's expected, every now and then. But you have to take care of you and your health first and foremost so you'll be able to be there for your loved one when they need you. It's easy to get preoccupied with the patient's health and what's going on in their life and forget about your own. You deserve to be taken care of, too.

8. Keep your humor. We all know Parkinson's disease is a tragedy and it's debilitating and, well, let's just go right out and say it, it sucks. But you still have to be able to laugh. Not at the disease, itself, but at life for finding it humorous to throw something at you out of left field that you weren't expecting. It might not seem logical to want to laugh, but if you hold nothing but anger, resentment, hate and sadness inside you, your loved one isn't going to be the only one who needs help and you won't be doing them any good, anyway.

9. Solicit help from others. Don't ever try to do everything by yourself. You may feel it's all your responsibility- especially if the

one with Parkinson's is your spouse- but you have your limits, too. You won't do anyone any good if you run yourself to death and hit a brick wall. There are others around you who are just waiting for you to ask for their help and when you do they will gladly give it to you, but they probably feel like they're imposing in your private matters so they don't ask. Instead, they wait for you to ask. You have more friends willing to offer you help than you can imagine. Take advantage of them once in awhile and take a little time for yourself because if *you* burn out, it's a problem.

10. Don't try to be a lone hero. Value others by allowing your friends and family to help when they offer. Remember that some people don't have that kind of luxury.

11. Don't automatically assume that you know and understand everything there is to know about Parkinson's disease and it's treatment. There is always new technology, new gadgets, new treatments, new resources, groups, Facebook groups like "Life With Parkinson's" (shameless plug) and a ton of information out there just waiting at your disposal.

12. Utilize all resources. There's a ton of programs available that are specifically designed to help those who are in your exact situation. Take advantage of them because that's what they're there for. Some of them might not be local, but that shouldn't matter because the Internet puts everyone across the planet virtually within a screen's reach of your needs.

13. Find a support group. More and more of these programs are popping up everywhere to meet the ever-growing challenges of an increasing Parkinson's population. They offer invaluable advice while allowing you to reflect, vent and share with others who are in your exact same situation.

14. Speech therapy. Since losing the volume of their voice is inevitable, you should plan ahead to ensure that the Parkinson patient will still be able to communicate and let you know of their needs. Although there are different options available, the best and most talked about program to handle that need has been the LSVT,

or Lee Silverman Voice Treatment.

The success of this four-week program is due to several things. For starters, there is significant improvements after as little as only one month of usage. Second, is the fact that the exercises are easy to learn. Third, is that you and the patient will notice immediate results as soon as you start the program. And fourth is the term of the success rate, which typically lasts for around two years after finishing the course.

How to tell if your caregiver is getting burned out

Becoming a caregiver is not something any of us set out to do. It sort of just falls into our laps when a loved one is diagnosed with Parkinson's disease. Suddenly, the entire household is thrown in disarray. The family dynamics have to be modified and the normal functioning of the household are changed forever. When you factor in additional expenses and the increased physical and emotional demand being placed on the newly-appointed caregiver, it can easily seem like a daunting task.

If you think about it, caring for someone with Parkinson's disease is like a double-edged sword. There is the part of it that is rewarding to know that you're helping someone you care about so much to get through this devastating disease as easily as possible. Then there is the unfortunate other side of it that is about how much of a toll it can take on you- both physically and emotionally. The problem is caregivers don't mind the second part.

Caregivers are angels whose selfless sacrifices can never be measured or repaid. They take on such a massive role of being there for their loved one without any thought or concern about how it is impacting them. Often, they let themselves go and jeopardize their own health just to get things done. But while we appreciate these incredible people more than they will ever know, someone has to look out for them, too, so they don't end up burnt out and sick. A caregiver won't complain and will likely run themselves into the ground without saying that they need a break. This is why it's so important that we keep an eye on them to prevent them from making themselves sick.

Caregivers have a unique role for several reasons:

- They are not paid for their efforts. They selflessly take care of their loved one without being concerned about compensation.

- They choose to do what they do. They voluntarily choose to be there for us, even though we never had to ask them to be.

- They are always "on call". They accept the fact that they are needed on an ongoing basis.

- They freely give of themselves and their time without question.

- They accept that they are in it for the long haul. None of us know what the future brings, but we do know that as our disease progresses, our dependence on our caregivers will continue to increase. They know this, too.

Since there are definite signs that your caregiver needs a break we, as Parkinson patients, need to keep an eye out for them:

- feeling overly stressed
- headaches and/or body aches on a regular basis
- overly tired all the time
- easily agitated
- feeling anxious/restless
- feeling overwhelmed
- unexplained weight loss or gain
- little or no interest in things they once enjoyed
- sleeping too much/too little
- feeling hopeless
- acting as if they're worried about something
- turning to artificial stimulants such as caffeine
- taking up or increasing their consumption of alcohol or smoking
- feeling isolated and alone

All of these symptoms will start to take a toll on the caregiver's health. By agreeing to take on this huge responsibility, they expect there to be challenges, but their bodies are not meant to endure such prolonged periods of these symptoms. After awhile, it all begins to take its toll resulting in a compromised immune system, an increased risk of developing chronic diseases and depression.

What can be done to prevent caregiver burnout? Plenty.

1. Have someone split some of the responsibilities with the caregiver. Taking some of the load off of them will mean a lot.

2. When someone offers to help out, let them. There's nothing wrong with accepting outside help.

3. Look for ways to help the caregiver get more organized. Maybe there are some things you both can implement that can make their job easier.

4. Make sure they routinely see their doctor. If they begin to experience some of the symptoms listed above, have them see their doctor immediately.

5. Join a caregiver support group.

6. Insist that the caregiver take time off for themselves- at least as much as possible.

Chapter 24

What Are The First Things You Should Do Once You're Diagnosed?

Obviously, hearing the news that you have Parkinson's disease is devastating, to say the least. You're flooded with a plethora of emotions and you don't really know what to do and where to start because you're too busy running off of raw emotions like fear, disbelief and shock. That's completely understandable. Everyone goes through that phase. But, believe me, it is just a phase because you now have a lot of work to do and the sooner you get started, the better off you'll be.

Once you've received the definitive word that you do, in fact, have Parkinson's disease, there are some things that you need to start doing immediately. Parkinson's doesn't take a break so neither should you. This is the quintessential example of "time is of the essence" because the longer you postpone doing something about your condition, for whatever the reason, the more Parkinson's will be more than happy to continue taking over more of your life.

Here are some steps you should take to properly start you on your journey to managing your condition. These are not in any particular order since different individuals experience different emotions at different times and may need to take certain actions before others.

1. Get a second opinion. As you read earlier, this is the first thing I did before I let myself be dominated by panic. I wanted to know, without a doubt, what I was dealing with. It wasn't that I didn't trust my first doctor, but this scenario is a little more important than, say, asking your mechanic's opinion as to whether or not your car needs a tune-up.

In my case I needed concrete proof that Parkinson's was something that was definitely going to be a part of my life for the rest of my life so I would know exactly what I needed to do. And I didn't just stop at two opinions: I got six. It might sound like overkill to some, but it wasn't to me. It's what I needed to feel comfortable about moving forward. I had to know and I had to know with certainty. Believe me, your doctor will completely understand that you want- no, that you *need-* validation from someone else to make you feel better about the situation. And if they don't, then you have the wrong type of doctor.

2. Try to stay calm. I'll be the first to admit that trying to tell someone who's just been given such devastating news to remain calm sounds a little more than ridiculous, but you still have to keep it together- despite your inner urge to go fall apart. You'll likely break down initially, which is to be expected, but you still need to get the initial shock out of your system and move on.

3. If you feel you have the right doctor to care for your needs, then start building a rapport with them right away. You're going to be relying on this individual for guidance in a great many areas of your life, for quite some time, I might add. You have to feel as if you can not only confide in them, but that you can trust them and their judgment in doing what's best for you. Remember: *they* don't have Parkinson's- *you* do so whatever advice they give you is going to directly impact *your* life- *not* their's. Listen to them and let them know that you're serious about taking control of your health.

4. Take a hard look at your diet. I know diet was covered earlier, but this is one of the single most important parts of your treatment. If you want to help minimize the progression of your disease, then you have to maximize the amount of attention you place on your food.

5. Get moving. This brings me to the next thing I wish I had known when I was first diagnosed:

Insight #12: The importance of exercise.

There's an old saying: "the three most important things about real estate is location, location, location." Well, I can take that a step further and apply it here by saying that the three most important things about treating Parkinson's disease is exercise, exercise, exercise. This is of the utmost importance in your life and is something that has to be thought of more as a necessity instead of a chore. It should be, without a doubt, your highest priority.

We're all busy so don't try to put this off by using the excuse that your schedule won't allow for it. If you can't do everything you need to do for exercise, at least do something. Something is always better than nothing. Even if it's just taking a walk, at least that's something to get you moving. And that, after all, is the key.

Before I get started, let me premise this by saying that every person with Parkinson's is different. Our metabolism, our body type, our genetic makeup, our muscles, stability, flexibility, stamina and age all determine what we can and can't do. I'm not suggesting that everyone immediately go out and start practicing for an Ironman triathlon competition, but the more you move and exercise, the better off you'll be and the easier time you'll have with symptoms.

As far as exercise goes, there are three areas that you need to focus on:

- Endurance. Walk, jog, swim, hike, bike, spin (biking in a controlled classroom on a stationary bike), aerobics, etc. Anything to get the heart pumping harder.

- Balance. Strengthening your core is essential to helping prevent falls down the road. Yoga, Tai chi, dancing or just performing simple core-building exercises will do. If necessary, enlist the help of a physical therapist in the beginning until you get down the routine.

- Strength training. You don't have to bulk up, but toning your existing muscles will work quite nicely with your balance.

Why The *Type* of Exercise You Do Is Important

We can all agree that exercise, in any form, is beneficial for Parkinson patients. But what if you have limited time, ability, energy, initiative or all of the above? In these cases, what types of exercise should you focus on first?

One of the best kinds of exercise for Parkinson's disease is aerobics because of how it gets you moving and gets your blood pumping. It also forces you to work joints that have a tendency to want to become stiff from non-usage. Since there's no such thing as slow aerobics you should see improvements in your balance, gait, stamina and motor functions. Some examples of aerobics would be:

- non-contact boxing
- running
- walking (at a reasonable pace to get your heart-rate up)
- spin cycles (stationary bikes built for speed)
- rowing
- swimming
- water aerobics
- elliptical machines

Regardless of what you end up doing, the main thing is to do something. Anything is better than just sitting around because the more you move, the less you'll notice your Parkinson's. Here are some exercise tips to remember:

1. Always remember to not only warm up before you start exercising but to cool down afterwards,
    too.
2. Know your limits before you start. If your body starts telling you that you're overdoing it, back off
    some.
3. Make sure wherever you're working out is a safe environment with no potential dangers.
4. Always have plenty of fresh water on hand.
5. Whenever possible, work out with a friend. It'll encourage you to go past your comfort zone.
6. Whatever kind of exercise you choose, make sure you pick something that you like so you're
    more likely to stick with it.

6. Pick Your Team

Anyone who ever wants to be successful has to have the right team working with them. This goes for everyone from a successful coach having the right team to a successful businessman having the right team. And if you're going to be successful fighting Parkinson's disease, you have to have the right team at your disposal.

Depending on whether or not you're able to consolidate multiple specialties into one person, your team should consist of between 6 and 9 people:

Neurologist. Out of everyone that you come into contact with during your Parkinson adventure this, by far, has to be the most important decision you'll ever make because there is so much riding on the type of treatment you receive from them. If you don't choose the right doctor for your own particular needs, you're only end up hurting yourself. Even worse is that your treatment and your quality of life will suffer needlessly.

Many patients choose their neurologist based on recommendations from others, which is fine, but you also want to base your decision off of who feels right for *you.* That brings up the next topic that I wish I had known when I was first diagnosed:

Insight #13: It's more important to find an open-minded doctor rather than just picking someone because they're "top of their field".

You can find neurologists practically anywhere, but that doesn't necessarily make them the *right* neurologist for you. There is so much riding on this one decision so you have to be extremely careful when making your choice. In fact, if you want to be honest about it, your very life depends on this decision.

Picking the wrong neurologist will certainly have its repercussions. It means that at the end of the day, your neurologist is going to close up their office and go home to their quiet, Parkinson-free atmosphere. Once you leave their office, you won't be on their radar again until the next time you darken their door for another appointment. They have the ability, no, the luxury, of turning off the world of Parkinson's disease and living their normal existence.

But as patients we don't have that option. So the few moments that we have in the presence of an expert on this condition are golden, to say the least. We have to treat these moments like we're receiving the secrets to the universe, which, in a sense, we actually are. That's why you can't skimp when making your selection.

A good neurologist should have a clear and thorough understanding of several important areas:

- neurophysiology- the science and study of the nervous system and how it distinctly relates to Parkinson's disease.

- Imaging- what types of imaging are necessary, when they are necessary and how to differentiate what the results indicate.

If possible (key words here), try to find a neurologist who is fully-integrated. This means that the doctor isn't tied to a specific hospital who is calling the shots for the doctor and making any final decisions on their behalf, which they will often do based on the hospital's budget or the range of services that they provide. That doesn't mean that doctors who are affiliated with a hospital are evil or sub-standard or don't have your best interests at heart. That's not what I'm saying at all. I'm saying a doctor who is fully-integrated has options. *Their* options. They don't have to dance to someone else's rules or comply to specific standards because *they* call the shots- not the hospital.

If you choose a doctor who is affiliated with a specific hospital, remember that when you choose the doctor, you choose the hospital, too. If they don't have a good track record, it might not be a good enough fit to risk getting involved with the doctor.

Also, be warned that if you go with a doctor who is hospital-affiliated, you run the risk of having unnecessary (and very expensive) tests performed, having tests unnecessarily repeated and being forced to jump through the red tape that is usually involved hen you're dealing with a hospital system. If this is all that's available to you, that's fine. There's nothing wrong with using them, if they're your only, or most viable, option. I'm just saying that it's nice to have a doctor's freedom of independence- if it's available. When their hands aren't tied, they can make decisions based more on what you need instead of what you're allowed, which provides you with a more specialized level of care.

When you first meet your neurologist, you need to treat it as an interview- just as if they were applying for a job because that's exactly what they're doing. So many people get overwhelmed and intimidated by doctors simply because they're so intelligent and they went to medical school. They put so much stock in this person simply because they have advanced education that they tend to treat all doctors the same.

It's fine to have respect for all doctors because they deserve it. I'll be the first to say that I have the utmost respect for doctors and everything that they have to go through to qualify for their title. But at the same time, you have to be realistic with yourself. Just because they're qualified to practice in the field of neurology doesn't mean that they're necessarily the right fit for you.

Your neurologist is applying for a job: the job of treating you. Make them qualify, just like you would have to qualify for a specific job. If you don't feel like it's a good fit, look for someone else- unless, of course, your insurance plan or your geographical location doesn't allow it. Hopefully, you won't become "stuck" with someone that you don't really connect with.

Get referrals. If you know other Parkinson patients, ask them for advice (just because they give you advice doesn't mean that you necessarily have to follow it, you know). Go on social media or on Facebook sites like "Life with Parkinson's", for example (another shameless plug).

Do some research. Once you find a doctor that sounds interesting, find out all you can about them: their credentials, where they attended school, what they specialize in and what types of patients they typically treat. You might find an excellent neurologist, but if they specialize in M.S. patients, that isn't going to do you the most good. Look at the Better Business Bureau for reviews and a history of complaints. Or simply go online. You can find information online (good or bad) on any doctor. Utilize it. If you can't get a referral from anyone, there are sites specifically designed for that sole purpose. Healthgrades.com is one.

Consider the doctor's gender. Not to sound sexist, but this does make a huge difference to a lot of people- whether they want to admit it or not.

Some people don't fell comfortable talking about delicate subjects with someone of the opposite gender. At some point during your treatment, you're going to come across touchy subjects that you'll be forced to bring up. You'll want to feel comfortable sharing and, most importantly, being honest with your doctor about them. If you hold back out of embarrassment, you might not get the treatment you need.

On the other hand, some people prefer same-gender doctors because they feel like the doctor will be able to better relate to their issues. And, let's face it: some people just don't get along with others. For example, you might find a male doctor who is highly-skilled with tons of experience, but who patronizes women and downplays their concerns. At that point, the doctor's training is irrelevant if he isn't going to listen to his patient and take her seriously.

Make sure your doctor listens. They might look you directly in the eyes and they might hear you, but are they actually *listening* to you? Yes, there is a BIG difference. When you ask a question, pay careful attention to how they respond. This will tell you volumes about them.

Are they patient? Do they schedule enough time for an appointment? If you call to make your first appointment and you discover that they're scheduling patients in fifteen-minute increments, my advice is to go somewhere else. This means that the doctor is more focused on maintaining volume instead of producing quality care. My main purpose of seeing a particular doctor is to learn what I can- not to worry about lining their pockets so don't be afraid to ask the receptionist how long the appointment will take.

Once you're in the appointment, you'll quickly get a feel of how well the doctor responds to their patients. If you ask questions and get short, rapid responses, it's obvious that they're trying to hurry up and get you finished and out the door. That's not the type of doctor you want to entrust your care to. Your care is important to you: it should be as equally important to them.

Another important point (especially in these days of escalating medical costs) is to know your coverage. Dealing with insurance can be a nightmare and often comes with unexpected and unpleasant surprises. Many times, insurance is a gamble of trying to find someone who's in-network, making sure costs are covered, making sure you know about your totally out-of-pocket expenses in advance, etc.

If you've been fortunate enough to find the right neurologist who's fully-qualified, has adequate experience, is on your insurance plan and has a positive feedback record, then you're up to the next thing I wish I had know when I was first diagnosed:

Insight #14: ALWAYS get (at least) a 2nd opinion or maybe even a 3rd, a 4th or as many as you feel you need to get in order to feel satisfied.

Nothing against your doctor, but it never hurts to have someone else's opinion- especially when we're talking about the quality of your life. If you took your car to a mechanic and you weren't sure about their diagnosis, you wouldn't hesitate to take it to someone else and get their opinion, too. You deserve the same kind of consideration (actually, you deserve *more* consideration than you would give to your car).

Doctors understand the seriousness of this condition. They aren't going to get their feelings hurt if you decide you would like someone else's professional opinion on your case. In fact, when I was diagnosed, it was my doctor who suggested I might want to get a second opinion. That doesn't mean I'm abandoning him. I've gotten additional opinions on things before and then returned to my original doctor just out of loyalty once my questions had been answered by someone with a different perspective.

There's something else that I feel I need to cover about your neurologist and that is that it's okay to question them. Yes, they are the doctor and this is their field of expertise. I fully understand that. But you still have to ask questions anytime they raise concerns. Just because they tell you something doesn't make it so. You can question their logic behind a decision and listen to their advice on where they're coming from. If it makes sense to you after that then go with it. If it still doesn't quite feel right and doesn't give you that warm, fuzzy feeling inside, then ask more questions until they have sufficiently convinced you that their course of action is the best option for you.

I'll admit, I'm hard-headed. My doctor has to convince me that what they're telling me is the best plan or I won't do it. If I'm not on board 100 percent, it's wasting my time and their's, so for the sake of everyone involved make sure you get all of your issues and concerns resolved *before* you leave their office.

One last point: it's always better to go with a doctor who is open to alternative treatment options than it is to stick with someone who only has a one-track mind. If the doctor is a "one trick pony" who only has one method and one method only that they never deviate from no matter how much you ask or the evidence that is presented to them, then you've got a problem.

Most alternative treatment options are things that have been in practice for decades- sometimes even thousands of years. They must have some validity to them or else they wouldn't still be practiced today, even with all of the modern advancements that are constantly taking place in medicine. Something has allowed these alternate options to linger through the ages. Could it be that they actually work for some people?

If your doctor discounts alternative methods then you'll be forced to make a tough decision because not trying something outside of traditional medicine means you won't be able to try everything that's available to you. If your doctor is dead-set on staying with just their way of doing things then you also won't benefit from the latest breakthroughs in Parkinson's research unless it happens to follow their standard treatment plan.

You need someone who is open-minded enough to consider alternative treatments that can even stray off the medical path of what is considered to be the "norm". Chances are, your neurologist won't completely understand some of these options, but that's okay. If you're willing to give them a try, your neurologist shouldn't stand in your way. After all, their primary concern should be improving your health by whatever means necessary- whether they understand them, or not.

Movement Disorder Specialist. Oftentimes, this will be the same as your neurologist, but this isn't always the case. Some Parkinson patients never differentiate between the two and automatically assume that all neurologists fit this category. But this is a huge misconception because there are some major differences between a neurologist and a movement disorder specialist.

A movement disorder specialist is a neurologist who, upon graduating medical school and completing their residency as a neurologist, has decided to further continue their education in the specialty field of movement disorders. This gives them an additional edge that a neurologist doesn't have.

Although I prefer working with a movement disorder specialist, I need to be clear about one thing: I'm not saying that there's anything wrong with a neurologist. Neurologists don't have to be movement disorder specialists to know what they're doing. All I'm saying is that a movement disorder specialist can have insights, training, expertise and experience in Parkinson's disease that a neurologist doesn't. And you can benefit from all of it.

After completing their additional training (which can consist of up to two additional years of study), the movement disorder specialist will work in a facility under the guidance of an experienced movement disorder specialist. This is their own specialized residency because it gives them ample first-hand exposure to Parkinson patients and the challenges that we face.

If there isn't a movement disorder specialist in your immediate area, ask your neurologist for a referral. Since they are specialists, you might have to endure some additional travel, but I'm telling you from my own personal experience, it's worth the extra effort.

Nutritionist. This goes back to that classic saying "you are what you eat". Parkinson's disease knows this all too well and responds to what you put in your body accordingly. There is vast amounts of information confirming that you can improve your symptoms simply by eating right.

Physical Therapist. Because Parkinson's is such a physical disease you really should work with a physical therapist (PT). Although most patients tend to wait until their disease has advanced into later stages to utilize the services of a PT, this isn't necessary since working with a PT early on can help you ward off the advances of the disease even more.

After a PT extensively evaluates you and your level of physical capabilities, they will be better able to customize a tailor-made regimen to fit your individual needs. This is different than enlisting the services of a personal trainer (which I'll also cover in a moment) because a PT is familiar with the effects and limitations of Parkinson's and can show you special exercises and techniques to stay as healthy and fit as possible, for as long as possible. They can show you the best and most efficient exercises to do so you aren't wasting your time doing things that aren't going to offer you the highest level of benefit as it relates to Parkinson's.

Occupational Therapist. Despite the name, Occupational Therapists (OT) aren't just useful in helping you perform your duties at work, although that is part of their mission. They also instruct you in ways to better handle the daily activities of your life from bathing and getting dressed to functioning around the home. They do this by not only teaching you helpful tips to accomplish tasks, but by recommending the proper equipment and aids that can assist you.

Speech Therapist. As your disease progresses, this is going to become more and more of a necessity. Even during the early stages of the disease, Parkinson patients can detect noticeable differences in the fluctuation and volume of their voice. When you have to endure both dysphagia (difficulty swallowing) and dysarthria (difficulty talking), sooner or later you're going to need assistance. A speech therapist not only trains you on how to effectively use your voice, but gives you useful tips on how to help conserve the voice you still have.

Counselor. It's always great to have a professional that you can communicate with to talk through your issues and challenges. While you can still do this with your doctor, family and friends, to an extent, a counselor is trained to hear what you needs are and extrapolate what is missing and what areas of your life need improvement. Just knowing that someone is listening to your needs is invaluable.

Personal Trainer. While they are not always necessary, they are beneficial, as long as you have the means to make it happen. Even though they are quite knowledgeable and we should always take advantage of that knowledge and experience, personal trainers aren't really there to teach you how to exercise. We all know enough to keep ourselves in shape- if we really wanted to. Personal trainers are there for support, encouragement and motivation more than anything else.

If you can't swing a personal trainer, always go with the next best thing: an exercise partner. They will force you to have accountability and having someone along while you work out offers just the right amount of distraction from the task at hand while making the time go by so much faster.

Chapter 25

The Importance of Support Groups

No one should ever have to go through a degenerative condition alone. We all love our independence, especially when we know there's a possibility that we could lose some or possibly even all of it down the road at the unrelenting hands of Parkinson's. It can be a lonely, dark, sinking feeling that no one deserves to endure. Even if you're fortunate enough to have caregivers to help you through, you can always use the help of others to give you an extra boost. Having this kind of insight makes support groups all the more important.

The main purpose of a support group is to instill in those with Parkinson's that they aren't alone. Support groups open up the lines of communication between people just like you who are going through the exact same things you're experiencing. Just coming to that kind of realization is a huge sense of relief.

It's very easy to feel isolated and tuned out from the world when you have a disease like Parkinson's- especially when you're first diagnosed. You feel as if no one around you understands what you're going through and, therefore, how can they possibly commiserate? You want so much for others to be able to help you but you also know it's rather difficult to ask something of someone when you aren't even sure what it is you're supposed to be asking. Plus, if you're like most Parkinson patients, you feel guilty just having to ask for help.

Right after I was diagnosed, I still tried to do everything myself (like I mentioned before, I'm rather hard-headed). I felt guilty asking my wife to help me with things so I tried to avoid asking as much as possible because I didn't want to burden her. I kept telling myself "this is *my* disease, *not* hers." I didn't feel like she should have to deal with it. She had her own life to live and it wasn't fair for me to put something on her that wasn't her problem.

I'm sure many of those who are newly-diagnosed feel the same way. You want to protect those that you love- not bog them down with even more problems. This is why support groups are so priceless. You get to mingle with others who are in exactly the same situation you're in. They know what you're going through and, out of everyone, they understand.

Don't dismiss the idea of joining a support group too quickly because, like you, these people are also looking for answers. Who knows? You might have knowledge or experience in a particular area that they need help with. Remember: it isn't just you who is looking for information and support.

If you are still hesitant to commit or you feel uncomfortable discussing your situation face-to-face with others, there's an alternative. Today's technology has made participating in a support group easier than ever. You no longer have to get ready, jump in your car and drive to a location. You can simply log in and chat with people online.

Conclusion

I hope the information in this book has been helpful to you. If I left something out, I apologize. I tried to cover all of the most common subjects and issues that we experience. My goal is to get the word out to as many people as possible so we can all live as healthy and have as full of a life with Parkinson's disease as possible.

I know I don't have all of the answers, but I hope that my experiences that I've shared with you concerning this disease will benefit you, or someone you know, in some way.

Remember that knowledge is everything with Parkinson's. There is new research being conducted all the time and many experts believe that they have learned so much recently and have developed so many breakthroughs that they are on the right track of discovering a cure for Parkinson's within my lifetime. I hope and pray that they're right.

I urge anyone who's not joined my Facebook group "Life with Parkinson's" to please do so. The members in this group are just like you and me. They love to share their experiences and knowledge with one another and I post news on it every day to keep people informed. I've learned so much from it just by talking to others all over the world and it's great to be able to reach so many others who are in our same predicament.

Stay strong and I wish you all the best in your fight against Parkinson's disease!

Printed in Great Britain
by Amazon